Mechanisms of Quality
in Long-Term Care:
Education

Mechanisms of Quality in Long-Term Care: Education

Edited by
Ethel L. Mitty

National League for Nursing Press • New York
Pub. No. 14-2550

The views expressed in this publication represent the views
of the authors and do not necessarily reflect the official
views of the National League for Nursing Press.

Library of Congress Cataloging-in-Publication Data

Mechanisms of quality in long-term care : education / edited by Ethel
L. Mitty.
    p.   cm.
Includes bibliographical references and index.
ISBN 0-88737-602-9
    1. Long-term care of the sick—Study and teaching (Higher)
Congresses.   2. Geriatric nursing—Study and teaching—Congresses.
I. Mitty, Ethel L.
    [DNLM: 1. Long-Term Care—organization & administration—
congresses.   2. Education, Nursing—United States—congresses.
3. Quality of Health Care—organization & administration—United
States—congresses.   WY 18 M486 1994]
RT120.L64M43   1994
610.73'61—dc20
DNLM/DLC
for Library of Congress   93-30194
                                                                     CIP

This book was set in Goudy by Publications Development Company.
The editor was Nancy Jeffries. Northeastern Press was the printer
and binder.

Cover design by Lauren Stevens.

Printed in the United States of America

Contents

Contributors

Sister Rose Therese Bahr, PhD, RN, FAAN, is Professor of Nursing, Department of Community Health Nursing and Gerontological Nursing, Catholic University of America, Washington, DC.

Ray Baxter, PhD, is Director of Living Health Programs, San Francisco, CA.

H. Terri Brower, EdD, RN, FAAN, is Professor of Nursing, School of Nursing, Auburn University, Auburn, AL.

Sister Rosemary Donley, PhD, RN, FAAN, is Executive Vice-President, Catholic University of America, Washington, DC.

Claire M. Fagin, PhD, RN, FAAN, is Interim President, University of Pennsylvania, and former President, National League for Nursing, New York, NY.

Gary Filerman, PhD, is President, Association of University Programs in Health Administration, Arlington, VA.

Robert Friedland, PhD, is Senior Policy Analyst, The Project HOPE, Center for Health Affairs, Chevy Chase, MD.

Pamela J. Maraldo, PhD, RN, FAAN, is President, Planned Parenthood Federation of America, and former Chief Executive Officer, National League for Nursing, New York, NY.

Clair E. Martin, PhD, RN, FAAN, is Dean and Professor, Nell Hodgson Woodruff School of Nursing, Emory University, Atlanta, GA.

Maria Mitchell, MS, RN, CPNP, is former President, Community Health Accreditation Program, New York, NY.

Ethel L. Mitty, EdD, RN, was Assistant Administrator Nursing Services, North Shore University Hospital Center for Extended Care and Rehabilitation, Manhasset, NY at the time of this conference and is currently writing, researching, and consulting on LTC issues.

Patricia Moccia, PhD, RN, FAAN, is Chief Executive Officer, National League for Nursing, New York, NY.

Bill Moore, MeD, RD, is Director of Organizational Services, Ross Laboratories.

Mary Ousley, RN, is Corporate Director, Professional Services, Hillhaven Corporation, Louisville, KY.

Rose Pfefferbaum, PhD, is Director of Gerontology, Phoenix College, Phoenix, AZ.

Peter Preziosi, EdM, RN, is Vice President for Executive Affairs, Planned Parenthood Federation of America, and former Vice President for Executive Affairs, National League for Nursing, New York, NY.

Catherine R. Price, RHP, RN, is Executive Director, United Church of Christ Homes, Inc., Hummelstown, PA.

Ellen S. Tishman, BSN, RN, is Director, Professional Development, American Health Care Association, Washington, DC.

Elizabeth Thornton, BSN, RN, is Administrator, Group Health Cooperative of Puget Sound Community Health Services, Seattle, WA.

Verle Waters, MA, RN, is Education Consultant, Dean Emeritus, Los Gatos, CA.

Paul Willging, PhD, is Executive Vice President, The American Health Care Association, Washington, DC.

Foreword

It is my privilege to thank everyone who has brought their expertise to this conference. At Ross Laboratories, our feeling is that the best return on our investments is to bring together the best minds—the thinkers and doers—to look at the problems that face the health care industry in the future. As a corporation, we can get very narrow-minded; not simply thinking of product development but losing sight of our customer base. A conference such as this brings us back to our commitment to being a partner in the delivery of quality health care.

Bill Moore
Director of Organizational Services
Ross Laboratories

I have been coming to these conferences for nine years and it is amazing to have watched them evolve into what they are today. This fifth invitational conference, Quality Mechanisms in Education, is a result, in part, of a recommendation which came out of the National Commission on Nursing. It is particularly striking to notice that we are sitting at this table about to talk about education, but with representatives from the health care industry, the providers. This group has become enriched to the point where we have some of the finest minds in health care participating at these conferences. The *quality of nursing education* is a new perspective for this group, especially since industry leaders had long argued that advancement in education was not well correlated with quality of care. Evolving from that short-sighted perspective has led us, finally, to what will be a much fuller, much more appreciated, and more profound sense of the need and the commitment to long-term care health reform.

Pamela J. Maraldo, President
Planned Parenthood Federation of America, and
former Chief Executive Officer
National League for Nursing

OBRA '87: Perspectives on Implementation

Presented by Claire M. Fagin at the National League for Nursing Long-Term Care Conference, December 1, 1992

The Nursing Home Reform Act of 1987 (OBRA '87) mandated a sweeping change in nursing home regulatory emphasis and is considered by many to be a paradigm shift in conceptualizing and implementing standards for nursing homes. After decades of experience where the provider was patriarch or matriarch in judging needs of the institution and its residents, the law positioned the provider as accountable for the quality of services, which in turn, the recipients (and their agents) might deem appropriate. It is almost conceivable that in time providers and residents might become partners in the improvement of quality care in nursing homes where they would be dependent on each other, accountable to each other, and equal to each other.

KEY ASPECTS OF OBRA '87

The Omnibus Budget Reconciliation Act (OBRA '87) signalled a change in focus. Key aspects were: resident empowerment through clearly stated resident rights; staffing requirements; interdisciplinary planning and care through a team approach; social services; freedom from abuse (which included the inappropriate use of physical restraints); and punitive provisions in the event of regulatory or health code non-compliance. It aimed to improve conditions of residents in nursing homes through the major change of placing in the control of the resident the means to reach and maintain an improved optimum level of physical, psychological, and social health. Nursing homes which do not provide the legislated stipulated quality can be removed from the Medicare and Medicaid reimbursement system.

Pilot Study: The Impact and Implementation of OBRA '87

Despite newsletters, publications, seminars and training sessions about the OBRA legislation, there has been little attention to the merits of OBRA '87 in what is called the "scholarly literature" since its final passage in 1989. To begin to find out people's perceptions on the extent to which OBRA '87 is achieving its stated objectives, I conducted a pilot study as a first phase in designing a data based evaluation of this important act.

The primary purpose of the pilot study was to (1) understand the issues surrounding OBRA '87 and (2) to gather data to inform decisions about the where, whom, and how of examining OBRA's impact. A multi-state survey will be the second phase of the study.

Forty individuals located in the Washington, DC area were interviewed. These people were prominent in decisions about OBRA '87, involved in its implementation, and held views of the outcomes to date. The resultant sample included current and past members of legislative offices who were active in the writing and eventual passage of OBRA '87, legislative staff who are currently "watchdogging" long-term care issues and promoting new legislation, representatives of advocacy groups, regulators, representatives of industry and professional associations, and selected members of the academic and professional community.

The interviews were conducted over a six-month period. An open-ended interview form was used to gather data. Questions focused on general impressions of the progress made so far in implementation of OBRA '87, where and from whom the respondents were getting their impressions, problems perceived at this time and predicted for the future in relation to implementation, and specific comments about the progress being made in implementing various requirements.

Data from the interviews were examined for themes that might provide for an appropriate ordering of the data. The resultant themes within which most of the views could be categorized are as follows:

- positive and negative feelings about specific aspects of the law and their implementation
- the survey process
- the cost data
- problems forecast for the future and chances of compliance
- strengths and deficits of the law
- meeting deadlines
- the place of long-term care on the political agenda.

The aggregate data from all 40 interviews are synthesized within these categories.

In response to an open-ended question about the most important single aspect of the law there was strong agreement that "Comprehensive Assessments" was the most inclusive. This requirement was seen as an overarching requirement under which many others were subsumed. The Institute of Medicine (IOM) also considered this recommendation the most important in its landmark work. A staff member of IOM stated that this was the only work they have ever done that was written almost word for word into law.

In answer to questions about the respondents knowledge and opinions on specific requirements, praise or concern was expressed most about reduction in restraint use, comprehensive assessments, nursing component issues including staffing, resident empowerment, Pre-Admission Screening and Resident Review (PASARR), and quality assessment and assurance based on interdisciplinary judgments.

There is a strong sense that positive change is occurring with respect to use of restraints. There is also considerable skepticism about whether OBRA '87 was responsible for what is happening in restraint use or whether the law accelerated changes already taking place. Workshops and conferences highlighting data from other countries and experiences in

the United States had started pre-OBRA '87. Word was out that reduction in restraint use may not increase costs; the movement was spreading
by word of mouth. For instance, the American Association of Homes for
the Aging reported that as of December 1991 their members reported that
use of physical restraints had gone down during the previous two years by
47 percent. This is an impressive drop and I believe it is unlikely OBRA
'87 alone had much to do with it. More likely it was the efforts of long-
term care professionals including nurses, researchers, and consumer
groups acting together, that caused the decline in restraint usage.

As we all know, the minimum data set system or MDS is the major
tool under the OBRA '87 law for documentation of the resident's functional status, physical and cognitive abilities, strengths, weaknesses and
problems. The main source of this documentation is comprehensive resident assessments, which as mentioned earlier were rated by respondents
as the most important single aspect of the law. Views expressed about
comprehensive assessments included concern about falsification of data,
problems due to poor educational preparation of surveyors and nursing
staff, contracting out of the nursing home for document completion, in-
adequacy of nursing staff, and lack of preparation of the interdisciplinary
team for their new or enhanced role.

Many respondents believed that good progress is being made and
that the MDS has a great deal of promise for improvement of quality of
care. Several observed, however, that the better the nurses and nursing
homes the less they liked the new requirements and the MDS, thinking
there was more attention to paper compliance than to real quality.

Concerns were expressed about the OBRA '87 mandate that every
nursing facility have a Quality Assessment and Assurance Committee
consisting of the director of nursing, a designated physician, and at least
three other members of the facility's staff.[1] Some respondents feel that
this provision is not yet fully understood by either surveyors or personnel
in nursing facilities. Several are doubtful about the eventual fate of this
requirement when 90 percent of care is delivered by unprepared people.
On the other hand it was said that the Health Care Financing Administration (HCFA) is working on this requirement, the social work profession is actively involved in helping with interpretive guidelines, and many
consultants are appearing on the scene to help nursing facilities.

Interdisciplinary work basic to comprehensive assessment and quality assurance appears to be very spotty with a wide range reported as to

successful implementation. There was broad agreement that personnel need more training in gerontology and geriatrics and in working together. For example, in many instances the director of nursing is a licensed practical nurse. In such cases nursing is lagging in being ready for interdisciplinary assessments. Respondents expressed a sense that increases in staffing were helping, that good will attempts were being made to comply with interdisciplinary planning but that there was little report of involvement with families, social workers, physical therapists, or occupational therapists in care planning. Further, the "sign-off" of the physician was seen to be a problem with physician participation.

Issues relating to the changes in requirements for nursing staffing and nurse aide training were given a great deal of attention by the interviewees. Concerns were expressed about the HCFA proposed rules on waivers for the nurse staffing requirement (or "non" requirement).[2] There is a widely held perception that the nursing staff requirement represents a major gap in the law caused by the compromises made in the committee in response to political pressure from several state government representatives and from the nursing home industry. There was a widespread view among those interviewed that in contrast to other pressure and advocacy groups, nursing organizations were not active in representing the need for nurses in nursing homes. On the other hand, pressures to minimize the nursing requirement were brought to bear for two ostensible reasons: the reputed nursing shortage and apprehension about offering locally competitive pay rates.

Concern was also expressed about the credentials of nurses in nursing homes, the lack of prepared gerontological nurse clinicians, the fact that often the only registered nurse is the director of nursing, the high turnover rate of nurse aides, and the use of "documentation nurses" to fill out forms (the latter concern came up in relation to many questions asked).

All nurse aides (or assistants) in nursing homes are now required to undergo specific training and testing, as a result of the OBRA '87 nursing home reform legislation. Costs for nurse aide training are covered, to a large extent, by additional funding from HCFA. There are many new programs and, it would appear, a whole new industry in this area that federal dollars are supporting. There is a mixed view on the quality of these programs, but a uniformly positive view about the need for upgrading nurse aide knowledge and skills. Two concerns appear evident on the part of the nursing home industry. One is that they will lose trained aides to hospitals. The other is the problem for those nursing facilities which lose the ability to do their own nurse aide training because of citations for deficiency and need for an extended survey.

Views about resident empowerment and the entire issue of resident rights were interesting and diverse. No one doubted the importance of the issue but there were major questions raised about the structure for compliance and the problems in implementation of the various requirements. The issues involved in resident empowerment are receiving a great deal of attention from ombudsmen and consumer groups. The law requires that Resident Rights must be posted in a visible, accessible location in the nursing home. During the Federal survey, the surveyors must interview several residents with respect to the facility's implementation of those rights. Several respondents believe that the requirements are too rigid and prescriptive and should not have been made into statutes. Others are concerned that the concepts are being misperceived and misused with the potential for abuse particularly in the area of eating and nutrition. There appear to be difficulties in definition and specifics of the law. The poor preparation of surveyors suggests to many observers that enforcement will not be effective or consistent. Finally, there was concern that the issue of resident empowerment might be out of balance with medical prerogatives and judgments.

Survey and certification were identified as major problem areas. Many respondents suggested that surveyors seem to have only a vague knowledge of the rules and therefore the results are subjective. Findings are not identifying deficiencies. Many believe that training of surveyors is insufficient (once a year); that surveyors' skills are widely varied; that there is no training or testing for reliability; and there is no evidence of monitoring. There was a great deal of concern expressed about the lack of a universal way of looking at scope and severity. On the other hand, there was the view that the survey requirements are a good initial step but it is too early to tell how effective they will be. Others were not impressed with using outcomes to trigger in-depth review and believe that the two-stage survey as mandated in OBRA '87 does not differentiate sufficiently. In general, the number of deficiencies are down but no respondent was able to explain this phenomenon.

Respondents believe the revised survey requirement would have merit if surveyors would be better trained and were monitored at the outset for reliability. Certain problems were highlighted, for example, that the "train the trainer" methods may not work; there is need for more surveyors; some states are working on competency testing of surveyors and there should be more; and relationships with industry militate against objective surveys. There was repeated concern expressed about paper compliance.

It was also felt that the surveys themselves were a problem. They are considered impractical, inherently subjective, and do not include longitudinal measures on dimensions such as mobility, weight, and activities of daily living.

The purpose of PASARR is to prevent nursing facilities from admitting anyone who is mentally ill or mentally retarded unless the state has determined that the person needs the level of services provided by the nursing facility. Respondents who were familiar with PASARR believe, in general, that it is well intentioned but extremely expensive and ineffective. A study done by the American Public Welfare Association[3] reported that the screenings revealed little which led to transfer or rejection. The screenings are labor intensive and use state funds that could be used for improvement of quality in nursing facilities.

Almost all the respondents indicated that there were no data that could give a reliable estimate on what OBRA '87 would cost to implement. Costs appear extremely uneven across states; some of the estimates have been considered outrageous.[4] There are no data to show relationships between cost, and reform or quality. The 1980 Boren Amendment mandated that long-term care facilities which operate efficiently and economically be reimbursed a reasonable and adequate amount. The nursing home industry has been slow in developing the expertise to sue the government but this step is anticipated from both industry and advocacy groups.

Many of those interviewed commented that the congressional budget office had done little on OBRA '87 and what had been done was underestimated. Currently, there are joint ventures doing costing analyses in more than half of the states but the information is not yet in. As has been indicated, the single exception to the lack of information on cost is the cost of implementing PASARR.

Answers to an open ended question about strengths and weaknesses of the law revealed agreement that the most positive aspect of OBRA '87 is the fostering of a changed philosophy for nursing facilities with a shift from institutional bureaucracy to a focus on individual rights and an orientation to residents, including resident involvement. Further, there was wide agreement that the overall law is very positive and the intent excellent. The mandate for comprehensive resident assessment is seen as a major strength of the law. Regulations on the use of restraints were also seen as very positive.

The questions about weaknesses or deficits in the law elicited extremely detailed answers, most of which have been stated earlier in relation to nurse staffing and waivers, specificity of the law, survey content and process, cost, MDS, PASARR, and the cost-ineffectiveness of the pharmacy requirement.

There was unanimous agreement that we are not meeting the deadlines set for the regulations and interpretive guidelines for OBRA '87. The major reason given for the delays (which, incidentally, are not seen as significantly different from other experiences) is the regulatory process itself. HCFA must reconcile the views of industry, advocates, regulators, professional representatives, and so on. This law has been heavily contested and HCFA has been flooded with comments. Further, OBRA '90 made some changes which brought previously issued regulations back for reexamination and redesign. Provider pressure has been significant. There was considerable agreement about the political clout nationally and in states of industry representatives in the nursing home area. Shortages of personnel within HCFA and the complexity of the process—the role of Office of Management and Budget (OMB), the anti-regulatory stance of the administration, the conflict between and among the players in the nursing home industry, the regulations themselves, the sweeping nature of the bill, and the prescriptive language were all seen as significant factors in the delays.

HCFA did not want OBRA '87. The staff believed that they were already moving in the directions proposed in the IOM report, that the law was unnecessary, and would prove to be excessively burdensome. Conflicts with the congress were evident at the start because of these differing opinions. Nonetheless, there is a sense that HCFA has made great progress with this law that has been more difficult than most in finding acceptable compromises.

In relation to whether the regulations are working and the eventual chances of compliance to the regulations of OBRA '87, most respondents believed that it is too early to tell. Regulations and interpretive guidelines have been late but there is a sense that what is out is working. Yet many states are asking for waivers and law suits are pending. However, according to those interviewed, staff at HCFA and in the nursing facilities are making major efforts to make OBRA '87 work.

In answer to questions about whether, in time, the law would be effective, respondents repeated much of what was described earlier: the law was too prescriptive and global; too many key people are unprepared; high turnover of staff militates against quality; and too many owners look at profit not quality.

Many felt that the good homes are being battered, and that the middle ones can improve with OBRA '87 but are not yet being helped in how to improve. There is also a sense that persistent litigation and payment reform will move the process along, but it may take years to make a widespread, visible improvement in nursing homes on the national scene.

LTC and the Political Agenda

The final interview item dealt with the place of long-term care on the political agenda. In general, the views expressed indicated that long-term care is not very high on the agenda and that acute care issues of cost and access will take precedence in the short term. There is great concern that the cost of long-term care added to health reform currently under discussion will have too great a financial impact for too few people's benefit. Further, once a "big bill" has been passed, such as OBRA '87, Congress moves on to other agenda items.

Other respondents believe that long-term care is a high priority on the political agenda but there is no consensus as to the incremental steps to be taken. Nonetheless, it is also believed that coalitions of powerful advocacy groups, notably the National Coalition for Nursing Home Reform and the American Association of Retired Persons, with various other advocacy and professional groups can push long-term care higher on the agenda over the coming years.

OBRA '87 seems to be a classic case of the regulatory process at work. Analyzing the law, the players, and the progress made are instructive and fit the literature descriptions of the "politics of regulation." As pointed out in Bardach's authoritative work[5], implementation politics are special, because there is an "already defined policy mandate, legally and legitimately authorized . . . [which] affects the strategy and tactics of

the struggle. The dominant effect is to make the politics of the implementation process highly defensive." Bardach stresses that the outcome of defensive politics is delay. And that is exactly what we have with OBRA '87.

How much influence do interest groups have in the development
and implementation of OBRA '87 regulations? Joshua Wiener from the
Brookings Institution has written that regulation occurs in one of two
models. There is the *pluralist* model, which says that all interest groups are
equal and contribute equal force in creating regulations; and there is the
political market model, which places most of the power to regulate in the
hands of the strongest industry interests. It used to be that the political
market model regulated nursing homes in the nation. The findings of this
pilot study would suggest that with OBRA '87 we have something closer
to the pluralist model. Notwithstanding the powerful influence of the
nursing home industry in delaying or even preventing new regulations,
the regulations for OBRA '87 are coming from the shared power of the
many interest groups.

Conclusions and Follow-Up Study

One major conclusion from this pilot survey is that further study is
needed to monitor implementation of this landmark legislation and to
identify problems in the interest of possible mid-course corrections. The
legislation was so sweeping that such corrections are inevitable, given the
interest in the field, and will be constructive if they are based on reliable
information. This study and others should offer regulators grounds for
investigation, discussion, and possible change.

I am currently completing a six-state survey on implementation of
OBRA. The states chosen were Louisiana, New Hampshire, New Jersey,
North Dakota, Oklahoma, and Washington.

Nursing facility administrators, directors of nursing, medical directors, other designated staff, as well as residents in three facilities in each
state were interviewed. Also interviewed were surveyors and survey directors, state and regional officials, and officials from state interest groups
representing providers, consumers, and the industry.

We do this follow-up study with a good deal of optimism about the
direction of change apparent from the pilot study. Despite the complexity
of issues and the political conflicts, there were positive responses overall

that are worth acknowledging. There is a strong sense that comprehensive assessments are a crucial process which is beginning to work and which will have an important impact on quality. There is considerable evidence that there has been a reduction in the use of both physical and chemical restraints. There is the belief that, in time, there will be a marked change in resident's perceptions of their rights to dignity, privacy, and care.

There are problems, but if we can identify and solve them and then build on the strengths of OBRA '87, these pilot findings suggest good fortune could be ahead for residents, as well as for the long-term care industry's long-term viability.

REFERENCES

1. I bring quality assurance and interdisciplinary participation up here despite few comments on this specific item because of its relationship with comprehensive assessments.

2. Residents in nursing homes with insufficient staffing, high turnover of nurses and related factors have been shown to have more negative outcomes in death rates, functional decline.

3. American Public Welfare Association. Medicaid Management Institute. (1990). *Preadmission screening survey results.* Washington, DC.

4. California filed a lawsuit against the federal government in March 1991 stating the new requirements would cost the state $400 million to $600 million a year. Known as the Valdivia Case, the judge ruled against California.

5. Bardach, E. (1977). *The implementation game: What happens after a bill becomes law,* p. 323. Cambridge, MA: The MIT Press.

Introduction

It is clear that the elusive phenomenon known as *quality* continues to be shaped by cost, ethics, social, and government or regulatory forces. And as these conference papers clearly identify, quality is—and should be— shaped by *education*. The participants in this Ninth National League for Nursing Invitational Long-Term Care Conference, brought together with the continuing generous support of Ross Laboratories, were prominent representatives from the provider, educational, professional organization, accrediting, and public interest associations. In short, they not only had a lot to say, they brought new ways of understanding the current relationship between education and quality. More importantly, however, they suggested that this post-OBRA (Omnibus Budget Reconciliation Act) era of health care reform being spearheaded by the new administration, in consort with health professionals *and* consumers, was a "window of opportunity" to create new ventures, models, and structures for quality in long-term care through education.

The goals and accomplishments of the first five-year plan of the NLN Committee on Long-Term Care (1982–1987)—"Overcoming the bias of ageism through education, research, and evaluation"—laid the foundation for the second five-year plan: *Quality in the Long-Term Care Marketplace: Indices, Costs, Mechanisms, Ethics, Public Policy*. This conference, *Education: A Mechanism for Quality*, is the fourth symposia of five invitational conferences charged with 1) identification of problems, strategies, and solutions for assuring quality in long-term care; and 2) suggesting recommendations to the NLN Board, committees, members and associations involved with the delivery of long-term care services. It laid the groundwork for a year of investigation and research into programs which exist, and models which should be encouraged, that speak to the principles, and deliver on the practices of, quality in education and care.

THE FIRST FIVE-YEAR PLAN (1982–1987): AN OVERVIEW

The first conference, "Attracting Nurses to Long-Term Care Settings Through Optimal Educational Experiences," was held just as the crisis in the shortage of professional nurses was beginning to be felt in all sectors of nursing practice: hospitals, nursing homes, and home care. It focused on preparing, recruiting, and retaining nurses—creating a career choice—for practice in long-term care. Issues presented, discussed, and published included: values clarification for long-term care; attitudes and humanistic qualities needed in caring for the aged; unique, meaningful learning experiences in the long-term care setting; the teaching nursing home; and the nursing curriculum for long-term institutional care. Collaboration between schools of nursing and nursing homes and the establishment of a "threshold curriculum" in gerontological nursing emerged as key concepts which could dispel myths about aging and help attract nurses to the nursing home domain of practice.

The objectives of the second conference (in 1983), working within the theme "overcoming the bias of ageism," focused on the nature of caring; courses, core content, and competencies in gerontological nursing; and gerontological nursing research from 1975–1984. Marketing strategies to attract faculty and staff to long-term care drew on some findings of the RWJ (Robert Wood Johnson) Teaching Nursing Home project, i.e., despite the negative aspects of long-term care (e.g., dehumanized care, insufficient professional staff, unattractive physical plant) geriatric nurse practitioner students spoke to the rewards and advantages of long-term care: autonomy of practice, the opportunity to provide continuity of care, and their ability to create change in practice and patient outcomes. The point was made, and it has been repeated in the years since then, that gerontological nursing has the potential to raise the status of the entire nursing profession. The burden of preparing nurses for practice and to "become the standard bearers" for the next century, however, was placed almost exclusively with nursing education. This responsibility, being better informed through understanding the realities of education-cum-practice setting, has evolved into a broader grasp of the issues and the opportunities, as the 1992 invitational conference clearly explicated.

Papers from the Third Invitational Conference reported on discussion of "state of the art" community-based initiatives in long-term care. The conference opened with a description of the prevailing roles and responsibilities of professional and licensed nurses, and nursing, in the nursing home. Subsequent presentations reviewed the known and growing needs of the elderly population and the implications for nursing with respect to congregate living, hospice, home health, housing, and nutritional services. Recommendations included: 1) the need to develop a model for continuity of care which included linkages for appropriate resource use; collaboration between providers from the various sectors (e.g., home care and day care); 2) development of a "user-file"; 3) case management; 4) continuing education; cooperation between the provider system and the education system; 5) measures to enhance and increase the visibility of gerontological nursing curriculum; 6) nursing participation in nationwide education to inform consumers about aging and long-term care options; 7) research into the use of available services and other services which are needed; 8) characteristics of the users; 9) values clarification for deans and their faculty, and for nursing directors and their staff, in order to look at the relationship between education patient care outcomes; and 10) collaboration within and between the various professional nursing organizations, and public interest groups (e.g., AARP, Gray Panthers, Older Women's League), and community-state planning groups—all of whom have a vital interest and role in policy decisions about care of the elderly whether living at home or in a long-term care institution. Appropriate reimbursement of nurses and the institutions in which they worked, marketing long-term care nursing, community nursing centers, and a shift toward wellness/prevention care were identified as issues which needed exploration.

Continuity of care and costs of care were the focal issues of the Fourth Invitational Conference: Models for Long-Term Care. The papers covered HMOs, home health care, a private practice model, and an intra-agency combined model of health services delivery to the elderly. The point was made that the richness of specialty education in nursing, occurring at the graduate level, should filter down to the entry-level and generalist practice. In other words, *therapeutic practice models* are needed. It was also noted, pre-OBRA's mandatory education and certification of nurse assistants, that continuing education for practitioners included the paraprofessional *and* that some content had to be taught "from nurses aides through the doctoral level," e.g., behaviors associated with Alzheimer's and related dementias; use of physical restraints; relocation trauma.

The Fifth (and final) Invitational Conference was on Educational Models, i.e., gerontological nursing and long-term care aspects. Educators and innovators from associate, baccalaureate, and graduate degree programs described curricula, models, and initiatives between schools and nursing homes. A critique of the extant graduate programs, masters and doctoral, was that none of them had a complete theoretical base for gerontological nursing. Lacking this, program evaluation is fragmented. As more doctorally-prepared faculty became available, a reasonable presumption was made that research into the learning needs of the students as well as research into the health care interests of the elderly would become incorporated into the curriculum. The clinical competency of nurses, whether they are generalists, gerontological nurses, or specialists, would reflect on the programs from which they graduated *and* on the measurable outcomes of patient care which includes patient satisfaction with that care. The papers and proceedings of each invitational conference have been published separately, by the National League for Nursing, and combined in a single volume entitled *Strategies for Long-Term Care,* 1988 (NLN Pub. No. 20-2231).

THE SECOND FIVE-YEAR PLAN (1989–1993): AN OVERVIEW

Fundamental to the goals and purposes of the NLN Committee on Long-Term Care, quality of care had to be linked to all aspects of long-term care and to education. Sound research was absolutely necessary to move information about care practices, the outcomes or quality of care, and education into public policy and programs. Accordingly, the First

Invitational Conference of the second five-year plan focused on *indices of quality through research.* The keynote speaker pointed out two things, 1) that if nursing did not address setting standards in an industry that consisted predominantly of nursing practice, then these standards would be imposed from without; implementation would be discontinuous and would lack an organized frame of reference; and 2) the standards should be "relevant and responsive" to patient needs; they should be "driven by quality, not financial, concerns." An extensive review of current research in home care and in long-term care (1984–1988) was followed by a review of research relating to outcomes of care. Complexities of outcome measurement and the rationale for using a conceptual framework were discussed against the background of diverse care-giving systems and staffing (classification and number) in nursing homes across the country. Environmental factors, organizational and social milieu, and informal care-giving services were analyzed with respect to quality. One outcome of this conference was the decision to conduct a Delphi study, in the next few months, on the nursing research needs of the next decade, the 1990s. The results of this study were described at the second invitational.

Mechanisms of Quality (Service and Clinical Outcomes) in long-term care were discussed by the participants at the Second Invitational Conference from their special perspectives, i.e., consumer advocacy and expectations, education, nursing and public policy research, home health care, and institutional care. The "Nursing Facility Reform Law," subsequently known as OBRA '87, was viewed by consumer coalitions and nursing service as a unique challenge and opportunity to creatively implement key aspects of the legislation: resident rights, quality care and assurance, and nurse assistant training. Discussion of the federally mandated changes in the regulatory and survey processes, paralleled by two new important sources of information—a comprehensive resident assessment tool to be used for all nursing home residents and Medicaid fee-for-service reimbursement data—were now available to assist researchers and facilities in outcomes measurement and the identification of quality issues. The point was reiterated that credible, usable quality assurance mechanisms were imperative; baseline data and thresholds had to be established. A quality assurance construct was described as was the mechanism for quality assurance in home care (i.e., CHAP). It was noted that *motivating for quality* simply does not just happen because it is decreed or even integral to the mission of the professional group. The methods needed to bring about congruence between the care-givers and quality-assuring practice lie in the domain of human resource management and education.

Results of the Delphi study found that there were seven categories of primary importance: environment; health promotion and disease prevention; patient and family; nursing practice; clinical problems; nursing administration and management; and staff and costs. Surprisingly, respondents to the Delphi study did not include several items which had national attention or were seemingly of enormous clinical concern (e.g., care of persons with HIV; incontinence management). The *research agenda items for the 1990s* in descending rank order were: 1) Patient outcomes (which overwhelmingly surpassed all other items); 2) Functional status: assessment and intervention; 3) Effects of institutionalization; 4) Safety features; 5) Postdischarge care; 6) Falls; 7) Depression; 8) Quality assurance; 9) Restraints; and 10) Sensory deprivation or overload. The "blueprint" for nursing research was established; now, it had to be implemented. A variety of initiatives were underway by the time the conference proceedings were published.

The Third Invitational Conference (1991) brought together representatives from the public and private sector to discuss policy initiatives related to the ongoing concern about quality in that marketplace known as long-term care. Very early in the proceedings and constantly noted throughout the ensuing discussions, it was clear that no definition of quality would be complete without reference to patient autonomy. *Empowerment* was as applicable to the resident's (formerly "patient's") quality of life as it was to nursing's actions to be meaningful. It was suggested that the "quality imperative in long-term care" should be based on the notion of "shared responsibility" between care-givers and care-receivers. The *lack of agreement about the nature of health itself* made the need to establish a dialogue between resident and provider even more vital—particularly with respect to establishing indices of quality. The "elusive agenda" of quality of care must meet the legislative mandate that nursing home residents should achieve "the highest practicable level of physical and mental well-being." If OBRA was to be a measure of quality, then training and resources were also needed; staff attitude and motivation were not sufficient in and of themselves. Discussion of future directions in quality coming from the provider community, included descriptions of private sector accreditation, pre-payment and managed care systems, and total quality management (TQM).

Although OBRA '87 was viewed as the impetus for quality, to one participant it lacked the vision required to move the nation forward on a national health agenda for quality of care. It was felt that the over reliance on high-tech medical care and the lack of a philosophical understanding of nursing homes and the care they can be expected to provide, required new approaches to the definition and assurance of quality. Description of the role of client/consumer as a *partner* with the provider in the search for quality indicators suggested that one could not only 'live' with the current regulations, one could go beyond them. This kind of joint venture can be meaningful, ethical, and have a secondary gain of shaking off negative public perceptions about the industry. One clear direction as a result of the third conference appeared to be an 'imperative' to think about quality as a component of *growth* and education. This thread, this enterprise, continued into the fourth invitational conference held in December 1992.

EDUCATION—A MECHANISM FOR QUALITY: AN OVERVIEW

The goal of the fourth conference was the issue of educational preparation of providers and the *role* that education plays, and should assume, in assuring quality in the long-term care *system*. Connecting themes from the previous conferences to the current one, a report of a pilot study on the implementation, effects, and problems with OBRA '87 requirements was part of the keynote address (Fagin). The study found strong agreement among respondents that the most important impact of the OBRA '87 legislation was the *comprehensive resident assessment*. Respondents expressed concerns about staffing requirements, education and training, and the quality assessment/assurance "piece." In discussing the relationship of quality in the long-term care setting to nursing education, Sr. Donley remarked that in order to evaluate education (process and outcome), one has to "know what the learners want, what the recipients want, and what the subject specialist wants." She suggested that educators and providers read a book written by an individual who had a chronic disease or disability. Presenting several different perspectives on the meaning of "quality," i.e., that quality is *the skillfulness of the caring action itself*, quality of care, she said, is also and fundamentally a "lived experience, a relationship." As "reactor" to Sr. Donley's presentation, Mitchell recalled the Socratic dictum that "a life unexamined was a life not lived." She suggested that the aphorism be applied to society (its health and social reform needs) as well, i.e., a society which does not continuously examine itself is not a society worth living in. Mitchell felt strongly that quality "is produced by an empowered worker . . . who has the authority to do what needs to be done and gets it done." This capacity is inextricably coupled with accountability to the employer, the co-worker, and the customer/patient/consumer. Mitchell also drew attention to the On Lok model of continuous care and noted the similarity between CHAP's ability to move the political process to get deemed status and the On Lok experience of getting approval for a non-traditional (and highly effective) health delivery system. For both of these presenters, as was well-discussed in their respective papers, quality was concurrent, ongoing, and active—not reactive.

Subsequent comments by the participants from nursing service and nursing education indicated their recognition that quality was in "the relationship" between care-giver and care-receiver. That being the case, the acute care clinical experience for students was too short. Moccia picked up on this point by remarking that today's students come from the "MTV generation": a five-second multi-image interaction between viewer and observer. Given that enculturation, how does one build *relationship* into the educational process?

The issues facing faculty in long-term care were extensively described by Brower. Faculty, she stated, are "one of the most powerful forces to potentially create changes in knowledge and negative attitudes in long-term care." Pressures on faculty and curriculum content come from multiple sources: social forces; technology; ethics; textbooks; litigation; testing; accreditation and state approval. In Brower's view, *a textbook is a social phenomenon and can shape attitudes through the delivery of information*. From Brower's perspective, the two strategic issues with respect to gerontologic nursing content in the curriculum are the faculty and testing. Brower has provided an extensive list of resources and references. Just after Brower's paper and just prior to Bahr's "reaction," the chairperson (Sr. McNicholl) stated that she had to interject (as a prerogative of the chair) that she felt now as she had felt twenty years ago, when she first became involved with the NLN on long-term care issues, to wit: that one of the major problems with reforming nursing homes and long-term care was that there were not enough nurses prepared in long-term care or in gerontological nursing—and that these people had to be "the movers and the shakers." She remarked that it was the people at the grass roots that had to implement the reforms and the lack of them twenty years ago is the same lack we have now—"the people are not prepared." Throwing down the gauntlet, McNicholl said, "What are we going to do, now? What are some of the actions that we can put into place? What is the planning that we can do here and now, take from this room, go out and try to implement over the months to come? That is the challenge of this conference."

In reacting to Brower's well-wrought paper, Sr. Bahr focused on the three issues which were critical, she felt, for gerontological nursing inclusion in nursing school curriculum: faculty preparation, school administrators (i.e., deans and department chairs), and testing for competencies in gerontological nursing in the national examination (NCLEX). She reported on a study of NCLEX test item content with respect to gerontological nursing content. Her findings were not reassuring. Bahr also noted that competencies of BSN and Master's prepared nurses have been identified by a panel of nurse gerontologists at a conference hosted by the National League for Nursing at Georgetown University in 1991 (See Appendix A).

Moccia's abstract, "Educational Advancement for Quality in Long-Term Care," contained the talking points for her 'plea' to the industry to give educators a place to take students where they can learn. But in Moccia's long-term care institution, it is a kind of social institution with new power relationships in a community of care-givers and care-receivers. Faculty, student, identified patient, providers, administrators, and community members as employees would become *learning teams* in a "learning organization." The long-term care facility as "nursing center" is a laboratory of nursing scholarship; it is "owned" by the learning team, the community. In Moccia's view, the issue is not simply to "change the curriculum" to include gerontological nursing content but to reconfigure the health delivery system such that the student (and faculty) are part of the community of long-term care. In reacting to this paper, Martin was not only intrigued but felt that Moccia's philosophy contained the seeds of a *culture for nursing;* we can no longer afford to have separate cultures for education and for practice if nursing wants to have a significant role in reforming health care. Martin brought up two issues which the "new community of long-term care" needed to address: 1) newcomers to the United States who are coming from diverse cultural and educational backgrounds and the women who will increasingly be informal care-givers to their aging parents and 2) nursing's need to engage itself in the political process to reform the educational process so that future faculty will not be able to fall back on the "fact" that students are not as qualified as they used to be.

As a preliminary to Willging's presentation, the commentary, assumptions, and recommendations in Tishman's paper, "Education Articulation and the Long-Term Care Field" were noted. From the perspective of the continuing professional nurse shortage in nursing homes, Tishman stated that educational articulation, (starting with the certified nurse assistant and LPN, up to and including the RN) is a valid and viable recruitment and retention pathway. The point was well-made that articulation models had to recognize work experience and competencies gained in the work setting, i.e., the nursing home. In Tishman's proposal, a key assumption of any meaningful articulation program must be one that recognizes and rewards education, experience, and productivity. Tishman outlined the basic minimum competencies that should be recognized in an articulation program such that the student might receive academic credit, waiver, etc. for same (See Appendix B). Tishman's paper—a description of the prevailing realities and real possibilities that exist in the current academic-institutional world, as compared with Moccia's "brave new world" of possibilities—included concrete steps that need to be taken in the development of a responsive and responsible articulation model. The role of the professional nursing organizations and their power as accrediting bodies was noted, as well.

As a representative of the provider organizations, in this case, the proprietary sector of the nursing home industry, Willging described the persisting negative impressions of nursing homes and nursing home care among the public and within the nursing profession. The myth persists, in all segments of health care and in the public view, that the industry resisted the moral, quality, and legislative intent of the OBRA '87 regulations. According to Willging, this was clearly not the case. The shortage of nurses, aided and abetted by erroneous impressions of nursing home care, places the needs of the chronic *and* acutely ill older person at risk. This is exacerbated by a growing shortage of nursing home beds. One solution, according to Willging, is for the industry to "home-grow" its own professionals by identifying staff who have the potential and interest to move up the career ladder. The industry has come to realize, albeit belatedly, that the complexity of care required by today's nursing home residents, requires the skill and knowledge base of a baccalaureate prepared nurse. Willging calls for a collaboration between schools of nursing, professional nursing organizations, and the industry to develop additional educational articulation models that accept and value work experience to meet part of the educational requirements for career advancement.

Representing a multi-facility corporation, Ousely concurred with Willging's report on problems with public perception and professional attitudes about the nursing home industry. She described a project at Hillhaven which identified effective, successful nurses (and nurse managers) in order to describe baseline competencies and proficiencies. This project is extending to all classification of nursing staff such that employees with career potential can be identified and motivated to begin their upward career track. Ousely felt that the concept of "differentiated practice" warrants attention, particularly in long-term care where role boundaries are blurred as well as merged between different classification of staff and level of education.

Unable to be present at the conference because surveyors were coming through the door, the abstract of Mitty's paper was the jumping off point for a discussion of policy and funding implications for education programs in long-term care. In the full paper, Mitty asserts that partnership between education and service (i.e., the nursing home) must be built on recognition and respect for the skills and knowledge base present in the nursing facility. In creating an articulated education program, Mitty feels that the school of nursing must have a thorough understanding of the kind of nursing home the school will be affiliated with. Numerous questions and issues are posed, for example: are the mission and philosophy of the education and practice setting congruent? What is the *degree of fit?* What *are* the competencies that each should expect of the graduate? Is the goal of the articulation the improvement of outcomes in the "real" or the "ideal" world? What is the level of faculty interest and preparedness; how is this determined? Has interest in learning and *learning preparedness* of the nursing home staff been addressed? Several proposals for funding education articulation programs—new or replications, e.g., TNH (Teaching Nursing Home), are suggested.

Filerman posed the question and restated the issue by asking, "How will nursing education position itself in the context of reform?" He suggested that the interest of long-term care nursing education lies in *structural reform*, in the issues of quality, capacity, and productivity of the health care system. Filerman discussed several premises of reform and described stages through which an ultimately integrated health care system will shift *from primary care to primary health care* as a central focus. In taking us through the parameters of reform—a most incisive, instructive journey—Filerman stated that the critical issue for the decade is "how best to invest human resource development capital." Nursing education is abjured to confront its problems, faculty and curriculum reform, with candor and with all due speed.

There was lively, if not intense, discussion between each presentation and response which informed each subsequent paper. An attempt has been made, in this overview of the conference, to include the substantive interchanges; they were informative and provocative. One theme which emerged early in the conference was that there needed to be a *change in social consciousness, not just in nursing education consciousness.* Everyone has to be part of the educational continuum: student, faculty, practitioner, consumer/patient, and yes, administrator. The suggestion was made that nursing education had to break the hold that acute care has on the nursing curriculum. While the hospital clinical care experience "works" for episodic care, it is not an apt model for long-term care nor does it speak to relationship-building which is at the heart of quality. Relationships take time; a clinical experience in a nursing home offers that time span, that continuity. The point was made that demographic data has identified growth in the population of the old (i.e., over 65 years) and the old-old (i.e., over 85 years) and that despite the obviously increasing need for chronic care, the growth in nursing home beds has slowed down. There will be more care-givers in the community, paid and unpaid (i.e., family). These individuals will need a "curriculum," also.

The question was raised that if we dispel the myth that med/surg nursing is the pinnacle of mastery and competency, what would replace it for safe, effective practice in long-term care? One answer was that community health nursing should be the forerunner of caring for the elderly in the community, but in education, community health nursing is hitting the same wall as gerontological nursing: fighting for credit allocations in terms of getting the time needed for clinical content and placement. Fagin reminded the conferees that several years ago nursing did break the grip of med/surg nursing—and moved the curriculum almost entirely into believing that nursing was an interpersonal process where "you didn't need to have med/surg skills." According to Fagin, this was an abysmal failure; it did not well serve the students. The students did not have adequate psychiatric skills; the students did not want to work with a really sick patient, yet, that was the only field in which they were at least minimally prepared. Directors of nursing in acute and long-term care let the educators know, fairly quickly, that what service wanted and needed was *a totally prepared practitioner*. Nursing education's experience, then, in breaking molds—shifting the education paradigm—brought them to the sobering realization that education had to provide graduates with "what they needed" for the realities of practice.

Several participants commented on issues and problems associated with NCLEX, the licensing exam, particularly as it appears to be a driving force on the curriculum. (Historically, the question items used to be based on what faculty taught; then, the exam became based on what new graduates were doing, i.e., where they were working within six months after graduation.) Moccia pointed out that the notion that the curriculum is the sole or predominantly responsible agent for students' performance on the State Boards is somewhat erroneous. Indeed, no other profession, including law and medicine, suggests that its curriculum prepares for the law bar or medical boards. To ask faculty or the nursing profession to become adversaries with the state licensing boards was not, in Moccia's opinion, the battle that needed to be taken on. Rather, she suggested, curriculum reform—nursing education—should be part of social reform. Nursing should struggle against "quick relationships . . . quick learning" and reflect, as had been noted earlier, that nursing *is* relational. Nursing has the "incredible opportunity" to have sustained relationships where the opposite is the predominant cultural mode.

Responding to a comment that "no test can be developed which is job perfect," the practicability of "computer adaptive testing" to replace (or be part of) the licensing exam was discussed. If the exam is testing "logic patterns," review courses would have to be taught differently because success on the exam would not be as content dependent as it had been heretofore. As we begin to focus on what the test is now testing, we would have to look for how we can prepare students to be successful. The impetus for curriculum and content reform came up repeatedly throughout the conference. By way of analysis, it was suggested that if very few new graduates go into obstetrical nursing within the first few months after graduation, then the number of "maternity care" questions on the state board exam should be reduced commensurately. If one applies that argument to why there are currently so few questions on gerontological nursing on the state boards, it demonstrates 1) that the "new-graduate-work-setting" rationale for state board exam questions is independent of curriculum, and 2) gerontological nursing will continue to be underrepresented on the state board questions since nurses who enter geriatric nursing practice tend to do so several years after graduation. (As a matter of fact, many long-term care institutions are hesitant to hire new graduates since the novice lacks the skills and experience to manage the complexity of long-term care nursing.)

The suggestion that each state have its own licensing exam would create hardship for nurses seeking licensure reciprocity between states. Rather than state-by-state licensing exams—based on vacancies, employment opportunities, and where new graduates tend to work—NCLEX could have special content "tracks"; the applicant/examinee would be required to answer all questions on "x" number of tracks as well as answer questions in the main core of the exam. The overall feeling among the group was that the usual and customary way of "doing nursing education" was no longer functional; the old paradigm of nursing education was essentially dead.

Returning to the issue of curriculum reform, faculty development grants for traineeships were seen as one way to acquaint faculty with long-term care in order to introduce (more) gerontological nursing into the curriculum, at all levels. The associate degree programs were perceived as being ahead of the basic and the baccalaureate programs in terms of the length of time and kind of experience offered their students in community health and, over the past several years, in institutional long-term care. Their curriculum included mental health and management courses. Waters described the nursing home-community college articulation, commitment, and capacity to identify non-licensed staff, i.e., nurse assistants and LPNs who have the potential to move up the career ladder. Faculty are "trained" to spot these talented individuals and to direct them to sources for guidance and support to enter the education track.

The cyclical shortage of nurses also plays havoc with curriculum stability. According to Fagin, and as she had noted earlier, nursing education is somewhat too responsive to the prevailing situation. Arguably, it almost has to be since deans and faculty hear from their students that they were "not prepared for what was out there." What is needed is a rational approach to prediction of needs such that curriculum can respond but certain fundamentals have to remain the same, i.e., the creation of an integrated curriculum and education experience in order that relationships and quality emerge. Faculty just might be resistant to curriculum change because it seems to be happening all the time; the content is barely evaluated before it is revised. And faculty are not sure what the curriculum is being measured against: NCLEX scores, positions available? One problem with adjusting curriculum to meet nurse vacancy rates is that the public data on the nursing shortage has some serious flaws. The most egregious problem with vacancy rate data is that hospitals are restructuring; they *are* cutting positions. Therefore, what may have been a vacancy last year is now a position that no longer exists, ergo, there is no vacancy.

Given the rhetoric about integrating health care systems, the fact remains that different nursing practice sectors are competing for students as well as staff, not to mention competition for faculty from the various education programs. A cautionary note was sounded: while trying to infuse education, quality, and status into the long-term care sector it could heighten isolationism and exclusionism between the sectors. What education *can* do, is integrate the sectors through the education experience. Case management could be a vehicle to build integrative systems of care and education. Filerman picked up on this; he stated that the nursing school of his dreams would be one where the core curriculum is *integrated managed care*. This would require that we reform the "specialist orientation" of faculty such that they no longer compete for time, space, and credits but, rather, they focus on the integrated care needs of the consumer, i. e., student and patient. There was unanimity among the presenters that long-term care must be construed as a continuum.

Looking at indices of quality, we should be evaluating different "transitioning points" in terms of the information which flows (and goes with the resident) from one level of care, or delivery-of-service setting, to another. At the present time, there is a major breakdown in this area and total lack of continuity. These issues were raised: 1) do our students, practitioners, and providers understand how serious this is?; 2) how much does this breakdown in information flow, this lack of continuity, compromise the quality of care *as well as* dissipate any nursing teaching that was done? Brower noted that if the curriculum failed to include clinical experience in the nursing home setting, then it was not teaching continuity of care. Parenthetically, it was noted that the physician, historically, has been the continuity-caregiver; in a sense, it is the MD who has been the case manager and has been with the individual through all the service settings. Yet, the physician role and responsibility as case manager has also changed, as a result of efficiencies which had to be implemented in the entire health care delivery system. Donley pointed out that it would be challenging to plan a clinical experience for students or a set of experiences for students in an integrated system; but the old models of supervision would not work. Attention was drawn to the On Lok program—a completely integrated system of health care where the staff works with the client no matter what the setting of care. Placing students in that kind of learning model could provide the relational and practical learning experiences our graduates require. Such a system might have the added value of reminding students (and practitioners) that care plans are still necessary, despite the fact that JCAHO no longer requires them in institutional care.

Total Quality Management (TQM) was suggested as a strategic new tool for curriculum building; it was a vehicle that might grab hold of a student in an environment of excitement and change around continuous quality of care—and relationships. From the perspective of the care-receiver, TQM is a completely patient-centered model of health care; it is completely focused on what the patient is, and what the patient's needs are. In education, TQM should focus on the students' needs; it should not be focused on the faculty, the provider. Mitchell stated emphatically that if the TQM system does not focus on the patient/student, the system will fail. At the nursing facility level, the approach to quality through TQM must have the complete endorsement and commitment of the senior leadership. Satisfaction with quality cannot just be with the identified "customer"; there are many customers in a nursing home besides the resident. Staff satisfaction should be another TQM goal. As part of a TQM strategy, articulation programs would be created between nursing homes and schools of education, such that nursing home work experience had some value toward college credit. Simultaneously, nursing home administrators and operators would need to think about flexible shifts in order for staff to attend school. Willging noted that career ladder programs for nursing home staff require collaboration between the school and the nursing home; each needs the other—and both have to bear some of the costs.

Mitchell suggested, as part of TQM or even independent of it, that nursing home managers need to expand on the corporate mentality, i.e., to move away from a single-minded focus on profit and loss to another kind of pay-off. Education has to help administrators and owners understand how to invest in developing articulation models, in "developing a long-range tolerance." Concurrently, industry leaders—the administrators, managers, owners—have to realize that there *is* a problem with education *and* that they are part of the solution. Education cannot fix itself in a vacuum; the settings of care have to participate in creating the learning experiences that the students and future practitioners need in order to make quality of care happen. Another key player in the delivery of a quality educational experience and in the outcome of care is the role and person of the director of nursing in the nursing home. It was pointed out that it is difficult to bring an education program into an institution if the standards which education wants to achieve are not congruent with the nursing department's leadership. Therefore, it is the nursing home's management, in the person of the administrator and the nursing director, which is a critical aspect of a meaningful education program.

To reach the preferred future, it was suggested that the coming year between this conference and the next one—*The Integration of Research and Education for Quality in Long-Term Care*—should be used to find the salient pieces in building a model for education of nursing students *and* staff in nursing homes. There is apparently a nascent piece of legislation requiring that every facility must dedicate a sizable percent of its budget for staff development and education; the timing, then, for a new model, couldn't be better. One suggestion is to take what has been learned from the community college-nursing home experience and teaching nursing home project. What were the structures, relationships, and staffing that made these programs successful? What are the criteria for success? Were the stated quality outcomes met? At what cost? The highly successful Project LINC (Ladders in Nursing Careers) in New York is an education-for-career mobility model that needs to be looked at, especially because it drew on cooperation and funding from facilities, the

State, and a major collective bargaining unit (i.e., union). Co-Op is another successful joint venture between home care workers and education. A by-product of the Co-Op project was the realization that an educated community of workers reflected the general community. It brings the notion of educating for social reform and reforming education into focus and clarifies goals. A strategic planning action plan is more than an exercise: it can develop a model, propose it for allocation of funds, use the model, and evaluate it; it takes a model and breathes life into it. There *is* funding for demonstration models; the rigor of strategic planning meets some of the criteria for a grant.

Interactive technology would allow video exchanges of program design, implementation, clarification, correction, and evaluation. It was suggested that our technology should allow us to pick and choose from the best courses in the country so that rather than each school using resources to teach the (same) course, the "best" educator/course should teach it to all, through the electronic medium. This has the added advantage of linking and relating the small, unique, underserved areas to the mainstream network. Interactive video teaching and exchange remains an underused technology. (As an aside, Filerman noted that no one should come out of an education or training system unprepared to work in, or be part of, an organized system.)

The relevance of NCLEX to what the education model(s) would be trying to accomplish and achieve, and whether the licensing exam would address those critical cognitive and behavioral factors on which the model was based, would have to be addressed. There has been a failure of the public, the industry, and the Congress to note what was achieved by the various teaching nursing home programs—why they have not been replicated by schools of nursing and facilities; why gerontological nurse practitioners are still not independently reimbursed. These are failures not simply of marketing but of vision. The proposal, then, at the conclusion of this conference, was to use the coming year to look for, and at, collaborative models between education and nursing homes. When the fifth and final invitational conference meets, it will reflect on what is available, and develop a proposal for a model (or models) that will move the nursing education paradigm so that it has the best fit with the continuum of care and with the delivery of quality in long-term care.

Ethel L. Mitty, EdD, RN

1

The Relationship of Quality in Long-Term Care to Nursing Education

Sister Rosemary Donley

The subject of this conference—the relationship of quality in long-term care to nursing education—suggests that if the linkages among these concepts are realized then the delivery of long-term care will be enhanced.

QUALITY

Although quality is a popular word in contemporary discussions of health care, it is rarely defined in operational terms. The Joint Commission on Accreditation of Health Care Organizations (JCAHO, 1986), the regulatory guru of acute care, defines quality as: *the degree to which patient/resident care services increase the probability of desired patient/resident outcomes and reduce the probability of undesired outcomes, given the current state of knowledge* (p. 11).

McElroy and Herbelin (1989) propose that quality in long-term care means: client satisfaction, efficacy of care, technical proficiency and performance of providers, accessibility, continuity, and cost effectiveness. However, quality is used also to describe the competence of the professional care team, the healing milieu, the food, the ambience of the environment, the care outcomes, the degree of regulatory compliance, the

1

level of resident/client satisfaction, and the enhancement of the life of the patient or resident. Schroeder (1991) synthesizes the ambiguity and elusiveness of the term quality: *Today's view of quality, then, incorporates knowledge, skills, and behavior of practitioners, as well as use of patients, physician, and payer measures of quality. Organizational culture, leadership, costs, productivity, and efficiency are also components. Because of this multi-faceted vision, the description, measurements, and ultimate improvement of quality are increasingly complex* (p. 3).

The search for a common meaning of quality is further distorted by the over-medicalization of health care and the invasive influences of the quantifying and regulatory movements within the long-term care industry. The media's ranking of acute care hospitals in response to the release of the HCFA (Health Care Financing Administration) mortality data illustrates medical influence on the notion of quality. It is part of our repertoire to speak of "quality" hospitals as those which have fewer than average number of deaths from any given disease. In long-term care, quality has become almost synonymous with compliance with an intricate latticework of criteria based on state codes and federal laws. When the Omnibus Budget Reconciliation Act of 1987 [OBRA '87](1989) mandated the assessment of quality as a criteria for reimbursement, it further legitimized the monitoring of such indices as: mortality rates, morbidity rates, failure to respond to rehabilitation programs, number of falls, incidence of infection, amount of weight loss, and the use of restraints. The nursing homes which are at the top of the quality list score low on these indices. That means that a nursing home with the least number of medication errors, the fewest restraints, or the smallest span of time between the evening and the morning meal is judged to be the best. Such a facility is presumed to provide the highest quality of care simply because it does not violate regulations.

It is unfortunate that *negative norms* seem to have set the evaluatory framework for assessing the quality of care of persons, because the absence of untoward events, e.g., accidental falls in a particular nursing home, in no way proves that the home is positively providing quality care. How, then, can we overcome the legal and historical reliance upon negative indices so that we can give a positive meaning to the assessment of quality in long-term care?

The dictionary (Webster, 1988) offers several meanings of quality: peculiar or essential character, a property or feature, a degree of excellence, an attribute, and an intelligible feature by which a thing may be identified. It seems proper to use "degree of excellence" to express an appropriate level of quality in long-term care. Classical Greek philosophy spoke of "excellence" as *arete* or "virtue" (Pellegrino, 1985). This notion has been taken up again by many contemporary philosophers and can be used to describe the actions which constitute relationships between persons in long-term care environments, in particular the relationship between the care-giver and the person in need of care. Excellence in long-term care, therefore, can be described as: *the skillfulness of the caring action itself; the good of the result for the recipient of the caring action; and the enrichment of the person who performs the action.*

Because excellence applies to interactions between persons, excellence (quality) of care cannot be judged by the economic or social standing, physical strength, mental acuity, or the political power of the persons who receive care. Excellent care must be extended to all— minorities, the poor, and those persons whose physical integrity is compromised, whose mental clarity is clouded, whose emotional well being is impaired, or whose spirit is depressed or inhibited. Excellent care is directed to persons, not to balance sheets, social registers, scores on resident classification systems, or investment portfolios. Quality of care must include human as well as clinical and regulatory parameters.

Assessment of quality and measurement of care outcomes should include positive signs and indices that good has been done for the person. Consequently, we cannot assess results adequately by merely counting up the mistakes we have avoided or offering evidence that no harm has been done. Excellence in results must be understood positively as an enhancement of the quality of life of the persons who receive care.

Excellence can be applied, also, to the assessment of care-givers. Every health professional knows the difference between the mechanical delivery of services and the giving of care which enhances a positive relationship between the person giving and the person receiving the care. A nurse or a health provider who gives quality care in a fully positive sense enhances the self and becomes more of a person.

In summary, quality care means care endowed with excellence in the act of care giving, in the enhancement of care outcomes, in the quality of life of the person who receives the care, and in positive changes in the personhood of the one who gives it.

LONG-TERM CARE

Long-term care describes a requirement for care which is continuous rather than sporadic; it exists over time. Long-term care is directed toward chronically ill persons who have physical or emotional conditions for which there is no known cure or consistently beneficial therapeutic agents. For many years, long-term care was almost synonymous with institutional care in sanatoriums or hospitals for the incurable, chronic care hospitals, and nursing homes. Today, long-term care describes a network and continuum of services which are extended over a period of time in the home, the community, the hospice, or the nursing home. When quality long-term care is the imperative, the three elements associated with the essence of quality—the caring act, the positive outcome of the action, and the caring attitude of the person who performs the action—are sustained in day to day experiences regardless of the care setting.

NURSING EDUCATION

The demographic profiles in the United States and Western Europe, coupled with shared concerns over health care costs, mandate the inclusion of information about aging and long-term care in the nursing curriculum. Where, when, and how long-term care material is presented and integrated with other curricular content has been, and will continue to be, debated in the literature (NLN, 1988). Several years ago, Brower (1988) classified gerontological nursing content, one major category of persons in need of long-term care, as normative aging, pathological aging, nursing, and policy issues. If the goal of the curriculum is to enhance excellence in long-term care, it is appropriate to emphasize a range of theories, experiences, and interactions which acquaint students with caring interactions, positive and improved quality of life outcomes, and models of service delivery which address the enhancement of the care-givers themselves.

Over forty years ago at the University of Chicago in a curriculum model now discredited by most nursing curriculum czars (Bevis & Watson, 1989), Ralph Tyler (1949) suggested that the curriculum in any field should reflect the needs of the learner, the needs of society, and the opinion of subject specialists. I will use his trilogy in discussing a quality long-term care agenda in nursing education because it delineates succinctly the areas of proposed curricular reform which, if carried forward, will promote excellent care.

Most persons who enter nursing school today (Tyler's "learners") have some personal knowledge and experience of acute illness, maternal-child health, and substance abuse. However, most of these nursing students lack familiarity with long-term care. It can also be assumed that many nursing students embrace the youth-oriented value system of the United States (Kuhn, 1990), what economist Uwe Rinehardt calls the world view of the "Pepsi generation." Repeated attitudinal studies of nursing students show that they lack enthusiasm for geriatric and long-term care nursing because it does not offer the glamour of intensive care or the emotional appeal of maternal-child health nursing. Conscious of the "needs of the learner" and the essential role the care-giver plays in enhancing the quality of caring relationships, curriculum builders are challenged to make the curriculum and the associated clinical and management interactions inviting, familiar, attractive, and challenging (Spier, 1992). The most innovative, informed teachers should be chosen to teach long-term care.

Health care financing and health care delivery reform are on the public agenda as needs of society. In a recent article in the *Washington Post,* Judy Feder, President Clinton's health policy advisor, wondered how a nation of 250 million people could spend $800 billion a year on health (Priest, 1992). Yet, if you look closely at the distribution of the health care budget, most of the $800 billion supports acute care. Nursing faculties teach acute care policy and financing in 'Trends and Issues,' and in Management courses. Some students are helped to see the tragic relationships in the clinical practice of acute care medicine, the behavior of cost-conscious hospitals, the level of health insurance within the community, and health care choices of poor people. As a result, contemporary nursing students are more aware of health care financing and policy agendas than any previous generation of nurses.

In the realm of long-term care policy and financing, however, there is private despair and public avoidance. Because long-term care costs are paid by persons in need of this care or by their families, these costs are not passed on in rising health insurance premiums or reflected in dramatic and escalating costs of acute care and high technology medicine. The real costs of long-term care are hidden from public view. The nursing curriculum needs to be expanded to take into account and make visible the financial underpinnings of long-term care policy.

A "reformed" curriculum will prepare nursing students for leadership in the delivery and cost effective management of quality long-term care, as well as for informed participation in public debate. To advance this end, students' theoretical and experiential repertoires should extend beyond nursing homes and examine long-term care networks in the home, in community-based services, in adult day care settings, and in other institutional settings such as hospices, acute long-term care facilities and rehabilitation hospitals.

Tyler also looks to subject specialists for perspectives on curriculum development. Who are these specialists and what knowledge about quality long-term care can be gleaned from these dialogues? Traditionally, nursing has relied on the medical and social sciences for its subject matter (Bevis & Watson, 1989). A variety of forces, the dominance of the acute care hospitals, public support for high technology medicine, and the power of state licensing agencies contribute to the continuing medicalization of the nursing curriculum and the health environment. It is foolish to suggest that the medical model be abandoned totally as a contributory source for the long-term care curriculum. Persons with chronic disease will attest that implants, chemotherapy, joint replacement, hormone supplementation, bypass surgery, pacemakers, dialysis, and drug therapy have extended and enriched their lives. However, because persons who live with chronic illness need more than adaptive strategies to adjust to the effects of repetitive, albeit successful therapy, the medical model is incomplete. Nurses who seek to provide quality long-term care need to experience the world view of the chronically ill, what Charmaz (1991) calls *Good Days, Bad Days*. They also need to consult with authors who describe the daily struggles and careers of persons with severe physical or emotional illnesses (O'Brien, 1983), (Guttman, 1961); and read poignant stories about living with Alzheimer's disease, cancer, AIDS, neurological afflictions, and heart disease (Stoudemire, 1983), (Ferrara, 1984), (Cousins, 1983). These moral narratives give meaning to the clinical study of long-term care and enhance the quality of caring relationships.

Earlier in this paper, quality of health care was said to be a function of excellent or virtuous relationships which motivate the act of caring, contribute to care outcomes, and enhance the sense of self of the caregiver. Ethicists and philosophers can enrich the long-term care curriculum by acquainting students with how the "good" or the excellent has been conceptualized over time, and by exploring the meaning of life and human experience with them. Nurses and other health-care workers who enter into long-term care relationships need to taste the intellectual and moral experience of the good and the virtuous. These reflections give meaning to their work and deepen their commitment to caring for others.

Another set of subject specialists, who can contribute to long-term care, design living environments and landscapes. Hospitals and nursing homes have chosen furniture, equipment, and designs which assist caregivers and conform to fire and safety codes. In the post-DRG (Diagnostic Related Groups) environment, even private residences have been arranged to accommodate durable medical equipment. The focus of design needs to be transformed to support caring actions, to stimulate positive outcomes, and to facilitate the quality of life and human relationships. Frank Lloyd Wright's (1960) insight that buildings should be planned to support and enhance life makes sense for the chronically ill because life styles are altered by chronic conditions. New ideas about the use of space, creative applications of color, light, and texture, and active involvement of residents and families will change long-term care environments. Students of long-term care should contribute to the development of these supportive environments.

This brief foray into curriculum building suggests that the needs of the learner, the needs of society, and the advice of subject specialists can shape the long-term care curriculum. It also suggests that schools of nursing can model new patterns of health care financing and innovative delivery systems to improve long-term care outcomes. This essay addresses the quest for quality long-term care from the perspective of nursing education. Education is an essential element in the tableau of long-term care reform because the outcome of education, in this case nursing education, is the development of informed, skillful, and virtuous care-givers. Educational reform takes on pragmatic meanings as well as moral overtones when it is recognized that today's nursing students, at the prime of their careers, will spend 75 percent of their time with elderly persons (Butler, 1980). However, reform of nursing education is a place to begin, not a place to rest. The demography in the United States touches every sector of public and private life. It is no longer possible to ignore the elderly, the handicapped, or the chronically ill. Public inattention, the absence of a coherent policy framework, and the lack of funding undermine and block heroic actions of individuals and make America less of a nation.

This paper began with a definition of quality and rooted its meaning in the word excellence. Assessment of quality should include a wide, rich scope of positive values. It cannot be limited to a calculation of the absence of negative factors, such as falls. Quality in long-term care is described in terms of the personal relationships between the care-giver and the recipient of care. Quality, therefore, embraces the skillfulness of the actions of giving care, the good results brought about for the recipient of care, and the enrichment which the care-giver experiences from the performance of genuinely beneficial care. A long-term care curriculum should encompass these positive dimensions and express them in the education of professional nurses.

REFERENCES

Bevis, E. O., & Watson, J. (1989). *Toward a caring curriculum: A new pedagogy for nursing.* New York: National League for Nursing Press.

Brower, H. T. (1988). An analysis of associate degree models. In National League for Nursing (Ed.), *Strategies for long-term care.* (pp. 409–415) New York: National League for Nursing Press.

Butler, R. N. (1980). *Why survive? Being old in America.* New York: Harper and Row.

Charmaz, K. (1991). *Good days, bad days.* New Brunswick, NJ: Rutgers University Press.

Cousins, N. (1983). *The healing heart.* New York: W. W. Norton and Company.

Ferrara, A. J. (1984). My personal experiences with AIDS. *American Psychologist, 39,* 1285–1287.

Guttman, E. (1961). *Asylums: Essays on the social situation of mental patients and other inmates.* Garden City, NJ: Anchor Books.

Joint Commission on Accreditation of Hospitals. (1986). *Quality assurance in long-term care.* Chicago: Joint Commission on Accreditation of Hospitals.

Kuhn, J. K. (1990). *A nationwide survey of student nurses' attitudes toward aging and their intent to work with elderly clients after graduation.* Unpublished doctoral dissertation, Temple University.

McElroy, D., & Herbelin, K. (1989). Assuring quality of care in long-term facilities. *Journal of Gerontological Nursing, 15*(7), 8–10.

National League for Nursing (Ed.). (1988). *Strategies for long-term care.* New York: National League for Nursing Press.

O'Brien, M. E. (1983). *The courage to survive: The life career of the chronic dialysis patient.* New York: Grune & Stratton.

Omnibus Budget Reconciliation Act of 1987. (1989). *Federal Register, 54*(21), 5, 358-5, 373.

Pellegrino, E. (1985). The virtuous physician and the ethics of medicine in E. E. Shelp. (Ed.), *Virtue and medicine.* Dordrecht, Boston Lancaster: D. Riedel.

Priest, D. (1992, November 23). Mixed signals on health care. *Washington Post,* p. A-19.

Schroeder, P. (1991). Improving health care quality in the nineties. In P. Schroeder (Ed.), *The encyclopedia of nursing care quality Volume I: Issues and strategies for nursing care quality.* (pp. 1–6) Gaithersburg, MD.: Aspen.

Spier, B. E. (1992). Teaching methodologies to promote positive attitudes toward the elderly. *Nursing and Health Care, 13*(10), 520–524.

Stoudemire, A. (1983). The onset and adaptation to cancer: Psychodynamics of an ill physician. *Psychiatry, 46,* 377–86.

Tyler, R. W. (1949). *Basic principals of curriculum and instruction.* New York: Harcourt, Brace and World.

Webster's Ninth New Collegiate Dictionary. (1988). Springfield, MA: Merriam-Webster Inc.

Wright, F. L. (1960). *Writings and buildings.* New York: Horizon Press.

2

Response to: "The Relationship of Quality in Long-Term Care to Nursing Education"

Maria Mitchell

The recent revival of interest in the Greek search for excellence, or virtue, as they called it, should remind us that the philosophers of ancient Greece also studied the individual to draw conclusions about what is the ideal state for government. In that vein, Socrates said that "a life unexamined is a life not worth living." Bringing this up to the present, we can state that a society that doesn't continuously examine itself is not a society worth living in. In reflecting on the keynote address and the study underway on the impact of the OBRA '87 legislation, I have to ask myself, "what kind of a society are we that we describe our achievements and our great progress in long-term care in terms of the fact that we no longer chemically or physically restrain our elderly?" As Socrates would say, I believe, we need to examine ourselves not to see how far we have come, but to see how far we need to go. Rather than be so pleased (or complacent!) about the very few positive aspects of OBRA '87, we need to look toward excellence and figure out how to get there, as Sr. Donley discussed.

The example of restraints gets to the heart of this matter—as well as to many of the problems in health care delivery—because the use of restraints was a typical response of the industry to ignore patient needs and do what was best for the provider, i.e., what was easiest to do, forgetting what the patient's needs might be. The new survey process, in effect as a result of OBRA '87, shifts the process more toward patients, toward outcomes; surveyors talk to residents to find out what the quality of care is in the facility. This is at least one step in the right direction. Unfortunately, most of the other regulatory measures of OBRA '87 fly in the face of what has been referred to as "positive quality," also known (for better or for worse) as "total quality management" (TQM).

At a recent meeting on quality in health care delivery, the economist (and social philosopher, I would say) Peter Drucker put it very simply— not by telling or asking providers and regulators as much as imploring them—*will you please believe that quality is defined by the customer*. Most of us discuss OBRA '87 in terms of its survey process and effect on providers. But what about the patients/residents? What about the programs that should be available to them? Where are the innovative solutions to these problems? I fail to see much innovation coming from the long-term care industry. We must totally rethink quality from the patient's perspective. Probably the best judge of the key determinants of quality is the patient or an active family member in a long-term care system. There *are* models where the kind of care and quality of care is patient-centered; the On Lok system in California is clearly such a model. In the On Lok model, long-term care is defined by the patient. The patient is provided his/her care where it is needed, whether it is in the home, in a day care center, or in an institutional setting; but the care is not limited to institutional care. On Lok staff work with the patient and the family to decide what is best for each of them; surprisingly, they do it at a lower cost when compared with comparable clients/patients in need who are not in the On Lok system.

The On Lok philosophy is very consistent with the CHAP (Community Health Accreditation Program). Coming up soon, CHAP will have the opportunity to assess the On Lok patient-centered model of care with what we believe is a patient-centered way of assessing care. A grant was awarded CHAP from the Kellogg Foundation several years ago. We were charged with the development of outcome measures for home care. Consumer input will be the fundamental source of data to define quality of outcomes. The focus of the Kellogg project is consistent with a patient-centered model of long-term care. Just as CHAP did, institutional long-term care providers need to look beyond the provider and regulatory groups for input and information about quality. You *can* get to concepts of "positive quality" from the perspective of the patient/client. CHAP's goal is the development of a system to assess quality utilizing *consumer-defined outcomes*—and to put these criteria into the accreditation process.

As Sr. Donley indicated, there is a need to define quality-in-work with a set of beliefs that are consistent with a purpose. The ingredients of quality require an empowered consumer and empowered staff, both of which are part of an administratively and financially secure organization. Progress toward consumer goals are mutually set. The entire foundation is based on beliefs about quality as determined by the consumer—in effect, the ultimate customer. While quality is the responsibility of management, it is every worker's job. It is *an internalized value* that goes wherever the worker goes. *Quality is produced by an empowered worker* who has the authority to do what needs to be done and to get the job done at the time. Coupled with this authority is the personal accountability of workers to their employer, co-workers, and the consumer.

Quality is a concurrent process rather than a reactive process; it is an active and ongoing strategy. Quality is measured holistically; it is larger than the sum of its parts. *The quality of the consumer's care has to be viewed in relationship to his values, his family, and his environment. Quality is the interaction between the user and the producer of quality.* Quality is the focus on the positive and the development of excellence in care-givers; people are the driving force of quality. If people do not provide quality care, it is usually because there is a problem within the system, not with the people. Finally, and not the least importantly, *quality should be data-supported, not data-driven.* Data should be provided for *learning,* and not simply for evidence that something has met survey criterion.

This approach to quality is patient-centered; it gets away from the medical model. And as you know from the On Lok model, this approach works. It is the responsibility not just of the long-term care industry but of the accrediting bodies to encourage and support such models of care. With CHAP, we are starting with the home care industry to encourage these kinds of models in the long-term delivery system. The same thrust should be directed toward nursing education in long-term care. It should be the responsibility of the accrediting bodies (schools of nursing) to foster changes in curriculum that educate nurses who are responsive to consumers as well as responsive to their medical needs. As appealing as high technology delivery of care might be, it may well be difficult to get nursing students to appreciate the needs in long-term care. We need to do a better job of educating nursing students—and recruiting potential students—about the social aspects of caring that are so basic and fundamental to long-term care. The providers in industry and the providers of education, and the accrediting bodies, have a responsibility to the public who are the ultimate users of the health care system *and* the education system.

Long-term care is not high on the agenda of health care reform. It is impossible to discuss the changes needed in education without discussing health care reform in its larger context. The fact that CHAP received deemed status through the regulatory process, and the Joint Commission did not, demonstrates that change really can happen in the political setting. OBRA '87 happened. It is not impossible, either, to change the N-CLEX focus on high-tech nursing. Empowering nurses in the long-term arena by, for example, eliminating the requirement for physician sign-off, will increase the visibility of nursing home nurses— through increased responsibility and authority (and accountability). This could have the effect of recruiting more nurses into long-term care settings as could shifting reimbursement from acute care settings to patient-centered models of long-term care (like On Lok). Nursing home nurses' salaries might be increased to appropriate levels—levels commensurate with their expanded roles and responsibilities. The new administration's interest in managed care is consistent with health care reform and the changing way of delivering long-term health care services. Reimbursement linked to quality outcomes may be anathema to the long-term industry right now, but rather than fight and hide from what may be part of a health reform package, the industry should move toward setting up models of delivery which combine quality care and financial responsibility. As the CHAP experience has shown, the regulatory and political stone walls are not so impervious that solid, informed, and creative battering will not wear them down. A key determinant in having a successful political process is knowing when an opportunity exists and acting on it before it is too late.

3

Issues Facing Faculty in Long-Term Care

H. Terri Brower

There are numerous issues that faculty must contemplate when consider-ing the use of long-term care in nursing education programs. Not the least of these issues is the faculty themselves, their composition, experi-ences, interests, and positions of power. Technology, as an issue, has tremendous implications for shaping and changing the curriculum. The use of required textbooks is symbolic of the relative importance accorded to a specific content area. As advance directives and other new content are added to the curriculum, ethics takes on increasing importance. Iden-tifying ethical issues as part of gerontological nursing content can provide legitimacy to aging content. Litigation as an issue is a concern that cur-riculum papers have previously overlooked.

Since most programs demonstrate great concern over testing and national certification examinations, no paper on gerontological nursing education would be complete without raising this issue. The forces of ex-ternal funding, accreditation, and state approval are all issues which ex-ercise substantial power over nursing programs. Lastly, faculty are reminded of the abundance of research opportunities that can be found in a nursing facility. Long-term care for the purpose of this paper, in-volves a continuum of health and social services that compensate the functionally impaired individual to maintain and adapt to limitations with the least amount of restriction. While long-term care takes place in a wide spectrum of settings, the term as used in this paper is synonymous with a nursing facility.

Need for Inclusion of Gerontological Nursing Content in the Curriculum

Nurses comprise the largest group of health professionals who serve older persons in the United States. Consequently, there is a substantial potential for nurses to have a significant influence on establishing and maintaining standards for long-term care (Tobiason et al, 1979). To a large extent, nurses' ability to set policy and establish high standards depends on their knowledge of gerontological nursing. Nursing education, therefore, could serve as one of the most dynamic vehicles for improving the nursing care of older persons.

However, the presence of registered nurses and particularly those with advanced degrees have been extremely scarce in long-term care settings. Among the many factors contributing to this scarcity are the low status accorded those who choose to work in these settings, lower salary and benefits than can be obtained in most acute care settings, a knowledge gap in gerontological nursing, and the lack of physician availability. The nursing shortage compounds the problem as salaries and benefits escalate in acute care settings making competition for nurses in long-term care even more severe. Even when salaries and benefits are equivalent between the two health delivery sectors, most registered nurses will not seek employment in long-term care. Contributing to the recruitment problem is the manner in which student nurses are educated and socialized in nursing programs. When students have limited to no exposure to the long-term care clinical site, they will seldom consider it a viable employment site after graduation. Recruitment problems could be lessened if students had sufficient positive clinical learning in long-term care settings. The nursing curriculum would also have to include additional specific gerontological content. *Clinical learning in the long-term care setting should focus on health maintenance, restoration, and health promotion.* The Community College Partnership Project provides an excellent example of the impact the educational process can have on the recruitment of new graduates into long-term care. The Partnership project led to a substantial increase in new graduates choosing a long-term care setting for employment. (While only 4 percent of the Partnership graduates accepted a position in a nursing home or convalescent facility in 1987, by 1990, after project implementation, this figure had climbed to 10 percent (Hanson & Waters, 1991).

The education process is responsible for shaping and molding the knowledge and values that students gain. How responsible has the nursing curriculum been in teaching gerontological nursing? Several studies have focused on the effect that the lack of gerontological nursing knowledge has on care provision. According to one study (Dye & Sassenrath, 1979) nurses had difficulty in distinguishing normal from pathological conditions in older adults, misinterpreting as normal any health problem that had its onset with later aging.

Robb and Malinzak's (1981) study found that younger nurses who had one or more courses in aging and were working in acute care settings were the most knowledgeable about providing nursing care for older persons. Sullivan (1984) found that *senior students ranked gerontological nursing content greater in curriculum importance and recommended that more content hours be devoted to gerontological nursing than did nursing faculty.*

Well's (1982) study of geriatric nursing care found that staff claimed their failures were due to short staffing, when in reality problems were due to a lack of knowledge and clinical skills in caring for older clients. When nursing programs do not sufficiently address the complex and interactive needs of the aged client, graduate nurses will not be able to deal creatively with the aged client (Rankin & Burggrat, 1983).

Further complicating the issue of gerontological nursing curriculum development is the lack of specific competencies for the programmatic levels of Associate Degree Nursing (ADN) and Baccalaureate of Science in Nursing (BSN) education. Verderer and Kick (1990) found that current literature for gerontological nursing curricula is limited primarily to general recommendations for course content, irrespective of level of program preparation. Because there is so much time devoted to community health nursing, leadership, and management in BSN programs, it may be more difficult for BSN educators to identify the urgency of adding more gerontological nursing content.

The Geriatric Imperative

The changing demography in the United States has been called the "geriatric imperative" and is a social and political phenomenon of immense proportions. The reality that the demographic imperative has not yet peaked for geriatrics (Kane, 1991) makes it all the more pressing to prepare nurses for the growing demands of an aging populace. The continuous population expansion occurring in the elderly continues to surpass projections for each census period. As a person ages so does the person's propensity for chronic health problems, health care costs, and the utilization of health care services. Health status data indicate that one out of five older persons has at least a mild degree of disability. More than four out of five persons over 65 have at least one chronic condition, and multiple conditions are commonplace (U.S. Senate Special Subcommittee on Aging, 1988).

Also, there are risk factors other than advanced age, such as the high correlation between dependency in activities of daily living and physical or mental disorders, which contribute to the need for nursing facility placement or increased home-based services. Gillick (1989) estimates that more and more institutional care will be necessary for the foreseeable future. The changes in demographics have resulted in greater need and consumption of health and nursing care by the elderly than by any other group. *Because they have special needs and utilize a larger proportion of nursing care services, the elderly should occupy a proportionate position of emphasis in the curriculum.*

Since many nursing faculties are not reacting to the geriatric imperative expeditiously, gerontological nursing faculty must become increasingly proactive. Nursing leaders in gerontological nursing practice and education can promote improved nursing preparation by aligning themselves with groups involved in aging advocacy. Community and state aging groups must be informed of the need to exert political pressure that would effect changes in the nursing curriculum. Older groups with political power could effectively lobby to mandate gerontological nursing inclusion in state licensing requirements.

ISSUES IMPACTING ON THE CURRICULUM

There are many pressures on the incredibly packed nursing curriculum. The faculty that include too much diverse content can end up with a curriculum that is fragmented and ineffectual. How, then, do we approach the multidimensional task of curriculum development and assure the right balance between the real practice world, futuristic concerns, current requirements of licensing boards, time constraints in which to accomplish what is needed, and the questionable ability of some entering students? How the faculty respond to including gerontological nursing in the curriculum will have substantial impact on where graduates choose to work, even years after graduation, as well as their specialty choice for advanced study.

Social Forces and the Faculty

Decisions regarding whether gerontological nursing is conscientiously included in the curriculum can be viewed within a number of contexts. Social forces play a predominant role in nursing program curricula. They operate in distinct and interactive ways as various groups, values, and beliefs come into contact and conflict.

The social organization of the faculty and their respective positions of power and status is important in shaping the curriculum. Within the social organization, faculty who obtain positions of power will have more resources at their disposal and more control over their own situation. They will usually be able to influence other faculty in the decision-making process. Small faculties may have less input than the administrator in determining the nature of the curriculum. Regardless of faculty size, the degree of leadership the dean or director exerts to influence the inclusion of gerontological nursing can be critical in assisting the often nominal numbers of faculty prepared or interested in gerontological nursing. However, the curriculum for the most part is designed and controlled by the faculty and is dependent on political and organizational dynamics, such as the interest and direction provided by the dean or director of the program.

Faculty themselves are one of the most powerful forces to potentially create changes in knowledge and negative attitudes in long-term care. They have the power to create change through purposeful restructuring of the curriculum to include additional gerontological nursing content, focused clinical experiences, and positive role socialization. The composition of the faculty, their specialty preparation at the graduate level and their relative positions of influence in the program have implications for role socialization of students. Faculty almost instinctively impose their own internalized values on the student body. The socialization process of student nurses can be critical in determining whether students will desire to work with other clients upon graduation or as an area of specialization in graduate studies. Bahr (1981) makes the point that faculty will not add more content until gerontological nursing is recognized as one of the "basic" specialities. Brower's study (1981) found that deans and directors rarely recruited gerontological nursing faculty for basic nursing programs. Edel (1986) had similar findings upon replicating Brower's study on a national level. Edel's study reported that only 4.41 percent of the 196 baccalaureate programs responding had faculty who had taken course work in gerontology and only 2.9 percent of the programs reported having the availability of one gerontological nursing faculty person.

Because the majority of faculty have received very limited content in gerontological nursing during their own basic nursing educational programs, they frequently do not perceive the necessity for focusing additional theoretical content on the aging client. Usually the faculty is comprised of persons educated in a variety of specialities with little to no representation in gerontological nursing. Since there are so few faculty and administrators who are knowledgeable about, or who represent a vested interest in gerontological nursing, their impact to effect change remains limited. There must be an adequate core of interested and prepared faculty to teach and stimulate interest in students in order to provide the focus and inclusion of gerontological nursing content for basic programs. Imagine a program without a qualified person in maternal and child health, or mental health nursing. Faculty vacancies provide an opportune time to obtain prepared faculty. The administrator must initiate a highly focused recruitment effort to obtain a prepared nurse gerontologist to be on the faculty. Realistic short and long term plans to recruit such a person will be required in light of the scarcity of gerontological nursing faculty.

Gerontological nursing faculty should be prepared with both a master's degree in gerontological nursing and a doctoral degree in nursing which includes a focus on the aging client. Currently, there are fewer formally prepared gerontological nursing faculty available than in traditional specialty areas. This reality is expected to last for some time especially in light of the low number of students nationally choosing graduate study in gerontological nursing (Bednash et al, 1990). When nursing education programs are unable to recruit a qualified person, the vacancy can be filled with a temporary (non-tenure tract) faculty member, keeping the position open until it can be filled by a person possessing the correct credentials. Fortunately, there are still a number of faculty who have substantial expertise in gerontological nursing and who were instrumental in early delineation of the specialty. Additionally, there are faculty who possess a certificate in graduate level gerontology, and who are prepared in the bio-psycho-social concepts of gerontology. Although they do not possess the more appropriate credentials, they usually demonstrate a strong interest in getting further expertise in gerontological nursing curriculum development and can be instrumental in creating positive curricular change. For example, *a faculty of 18 should have at least three persons who can represent gerontological nursing.* At least one of the three should have the appropriate credentials, as described above.

If it is unrealistic to recruit gerontological nursing faculty, such as for a small tenured faculty where little turnover is expected, other measures can be taken. The faculty and administrator could decide to develop a home-grown faculty person who, in turn, will assist in "gerontologizing" the entire faculty. This process of socializing an entire faculty would be facilitated by extramural monies to give identified faculty members time to acquire the necessary expertise. Recent literature documents that there has been progress in obtaining prepared faculty or in developing those already on the faculty (Malliarakis and Heine, 1990). Although most authors have focused on the lack of prepared faculty, more faculty are now indicating that they received some formal content in their basic programs. The recently completed Southern Regional Educational Board's (SREB) study of 231 nursing programs found that about 12 percent of faculty in the Southern region report some preparation in gerontological nursing (Yurchuck & Brower, 1992).

Technology in the Curriculum

A second issue, the rising complexity of technological advances, has catapulted nursing practice and education into the age of computerization. Interactive videos and computer assisted instruction are already available in the majority of specialty areas as a host of subject areas. However, computer aides in gerontological nursing remain scarce, leaving ample room for development.

Health care technological advances have resulted in an increase in life span and rising number of chronic health problems in the elderly. Another hazard of technological wizardry is the concomitant increase in the acuity level of clients and increased intensity of health care services in all settings. That increase is particularly prevalent in tertiary health care centers. Technological advances mean that highly educated nurses must learn to interact with sophisticated equipment. This has led to a greater emphasis in the nursing curriculum on the acutely ill client or intensive care nursing. Faculty are cautioned against designing a curriculum that reflects an overriding emphasis on acute care nursing, to the neglect of other areas, as the health marketplace is growing more rapidly in the long-term care health field.

Nursing students respond to the challenges of complex technology and feel the need to master them. They wish to gain as much experience with acutely ill clients as possible while they are still students; they are not eager to deal with clients who have a chronic illness. Responding to re-cruiting pressures of health centers and student interest, many nursing programs now offer a course on care of the client with "complex nursing needs" or, in other words, a course where clinical experiences are ob-tained in intensive care nursing units. At one school, the complex nurs-ing needs course was provided at the same time as the gerontological nursing course. Students focused their studies on the complex care course, and some openly admitted that since they intended to work in a critical care area after graduation, they intentionally neglected studying for the gerontological nursing course. However, many faculty would be surprised to learn that nursing facilities are having to deal with increased intensity of nursing services and many have created special care units (SCU). The ventilator, AIDS, and Alzheimer's SCUs in the long-term care facility lend themselves to student clinicals that reflect more inten-sive nursing services (Bauer & Roedel, 1992). Furthermore, more and more health care centers are recognizing the marketability of geriatric services and are opening skilled nursing care units and other services geared to older clients.

Ethics in the Curriculum

Another potential influence on the curriculum is the increasing emphasis on ethical dilemmas for such topics as active or passive euthanasia, owner-ship of fertilized ova, advance directives, patient care rights, and the ra-tioning of health care resources. Ethical concerns are being included in the nursing curriculum and rightfully should be addressed. Of utmost importance, however, is that while ethical concerns should cover the life span, care should be taken to insure that they include pertinent and age specific aspects focused on older clients.

Many older persons confuse the issue of advance directives with the limiting of health care resources and are unaware that, in actuality, an advance directive will empower them with the right to a choice. The current movement to limit restraint use has caused many nurses to consider the ethical dilemmas of using restraints. Included in a discussion of the ethical dimensions regarding restraints, for example, are considerations for human rights, quality of life issues, competency, the right to fall with its potential for injury in exchange for freedom, restorative nursing versus debilitating persons by tying them down, and issues of decision making. Students need to be attuned to these and other ethical issues in order to assist the elderly in dealing with ethical problems. Ethics is only one of many subjects where the elderly can be emphasized. Bahr (1992) makes the case for ethical practice of nursing care of the older person. She points out that *a nurse will have difficulty in carrying out the principle of beneficence if the nurse does not have sufficient knowledge to recognize atypical presentations of health problems.*

Textbooks

The importance of textbooks *as a social phenomenon* should not be underestimated, but is frequently overlooked when discussing how the curriculum is influenced. Faculty select readings and require textbooks that reinforce their beliefs and attitudes regarding what students need to know. The textbook holds unparalled importance in influencing what will be taught in the nursing curriculum. Texts provide a level of content expertise that few faculty possess. Texts also influence how topics will be regarded or the value we place on that content. The SREB (1991) study of nursing programs in 18 regional southern states found that only 20 percent required a gerontological nursing text. Even when a required course in gerontological nursing is improbable, students should be required to purchase a textbook, just as they do for community health, mental health, child health, etc. Unfortunately, the high costs of texts leads many nursing faculty to decide on fewer required books. In that case, faculty should select the best texts available that include the most current content on the older adult. But when there is no required course, the mere requiring of a textbook will not insure that the text is used appropriately throughout the curriculum. A required text can serve as a token that is seldom used.

Litigation

Legal issues and court decisions that grow out of litigation are two forces that have the potential for influencing the nursing curriculum. Increasingly, the concern for quality assurance has come about with institutions being held accountable for meeting standards of care through the vehicle of legal action. A large proportion of legal cases involve the older client. Nursing faculty would be wise to keep abreast of the cases that are in the court system, giving particular attention to the standards of care that are being abridged, and the common law that is evolving out of litigation. Then, the curriculum could be adjusted to ensure that prevention of negligence suits is directed through educational design and not legal precedent. Including the American Nurses Association Standards of Gerontological Nursing Practice in the curriculum provides students with national standards as criteria for practice that hold up under intensive legal scrutiny.

Testing

The measuring of performance through testing in the curriculum and licensing examinations are perhaps the most vital issues that influence the nursing curriculum. The choice and number of text questions on specified content are perceived by students as content that faculty value and have significance in the curriculum. There should be increased gerontological testing in the curriculum that is age and content specific, or proportionate to the real practice world where graduates will eventually be practicing nursing.

Faculty's concern with measured performance validates the impact that licensing examinations have on the curriculum. The licensing examination profoundly influences the ways in which nursing schools function. That influence is particularly strong in directing revisions of the curriculum. Licensing examinations are geared to hospital nursing and neglect the older client and long-term care nursing found in both home health care and nursing facilities. Rayfield (1990), a national consultant and provider of the NCLEX-RN review workshops, analyzed NCLEX test content, according to frequency and criticality or the weighing of importance of items. She noted that criticality of activities ranges from a score of .08 to 3.46. A comparison of criticality scores between maternal and infant health and gerontological nursing reveals that there are 11 activities associated with maternal and child health for a total criticality score of 4.98. There are only three activities that can be identified as closest to gerontological nursing content: plan a bowel or bladder retraining program, help a client to perform activities of daily living, and counsel a client with urinary or bowel incontinence. The total criticality score is 2.75. Echoing Rayfield's analysis of NCLEX is Arnett's computerized programs to assist students and graduates prepare for the licensing examination. Arnett's computer discs provide 800 questions for pre/post testing in pediatrics, obstetrics, psychiatric, and medical-surgical. There is no mention of gerontological nursing.

The most realistic deterrent to the inclusion of additional gerontological nursing theory and practice in long-term care continues to be the lack of accountability on the testing of that content in the current NCLEX examination. NCLEX *must* include specific questions on long-term care if the teaching of long-term care is to be legitimized in the nursing curriculum. *If the nursing licensing examination reported on more discrete content areas, such as the percentage of questions involving older clients and resultant graduate success rate, it would be easier to spot curricular deficiencies.* The political levers of state and federal regulations would produce a greater emphasis in gerontological nursing testing on the licensing examination.

External Funding

The external forces of extramural funding has brought about a modicum of change for a small number of nursing programs. Both federal and private foundations have exerted substantial influence in bringing about positive change to include greater attention to long-term care and the older client. The Division of Nursing Special Projects has brought about substantial change in individual schools and whole regions. Unfortunately, curriculum projects for either the integration of content or continuing education is no longer considered by Congress a target for fundable Special Nursing Projects, in spite of the reality that there continues to be a great need. The Robert Wood Johnson (RWJ) and the Kellogg Foundation have also provided substantial support and continue to provide support in the form of different projects. The RWJ Teaching Nursing Home projects produced commendable results for the small number of BSN programs that were included in funding. The dissemination of publishing and media production of results should have some impact on encouraging other programs to attempt similar endeavors. The Community College Nursing Home Partnership Project, funded by the Kellogg Foundation, has been the most promising development in the field of delineating gerontological nursing curriculum for ADN education. The Partnership project has had substantial impact on the caregiving by nursing staff in the nursing homes sites. Registered nurses performed more comprehensive physical assessments and increased their identification of residents' needs. Nurses also increased restorative nursing and documentation, indicating that care was more individualized (Carignan, 1992).

Accreditation and State Approval

The external forces of the accrediting and state board approval bodies have the potential to exert far more influence than is evident. They could insure that gerontological nursing is adequately and appropriately addressed in the nursing curriculum. Can anyone imagine a program being accredited or receiving state approval without sufficient theoretical content and clinical practice in maternal and infant or child health nursing? While *a few states now mandate inclusion of gerontological nursing in some fashion*, the large majority do not recognize the validity of a regulation that would single out one content area. Even in states where there are state mandates to include gerontological nursing, the state board of nursing has often laxly interpreted the rules and regulations to conclude that evidence of clinical exposure to the older client is sufficient. At least one state board of nursing actually discouraged any additional focus in gerontological nursing (Brower, 1988).

The National League for Nursing has the potential for exerting pressure to include more gerontological nursing content and emphasis on long-term care nursing. While no accreditation criteria specifically speaks to gerontological nursing content, a criterion calling for provision of the theoretical and clinical caring activities for clients across the life span implies that the curriculum should contain some gerontological nursing content. The use of more site visitors who have expertise in gerontological nursing could provide one means of subtle pressure in lieu of a specific criterion. Clearly, there is a lack of progress to make inclusion mandatory. Multiple forces interact to mitigate against greater inclusion or emphasis on gerontological nursing in the curriculum. Because of this reality, the elderly go on receiving less than adequate care by nurses who lack a sufficient knowledge base. Again, state and federal regulations may be required to exert sufficient pressure on state boards of nursing and NCLEX examinations to add additional emphasis to long-term care and gerontological nursing test items.

Research Opportunities

The long-term care setting provides faculty with a natural laboratory to conduct a wide variety of research projects. Faculty interested in managerial aspects will find a fertile field in the nursing facility setting. Questions related to policy setting for long-term care will enable faculty to broaden their views of health care in America. Research on clinical subjects is time consuming regardless of the setting, but can be even more problematic in the long-term care setting. The necessity of signed consents that involves contact with guardians has frequently discouraged all but the most seasoned researcher. In spite of that obstacle, faculty will find most nursing facility personnel eager to assist and facilitate the research process in any way that they can. More nursing facilities have created an 'institutional review board,' but gaining access still remains easier than the larger health centers.

Conclusion

In sum, this discussion of issues should not be considered all inclusive of relevant and important issues that effect successful and increased inclusion of gerontological nursing and long-term care. The two most strategic issues relate to the faculty themselves and testing. The faculty organization needs to have representative gerontological faculty, either through recruitment or development activities. The nursing facility presents many challenges for novice and experienced faculty alike. Not the least of those challenges is the attitudes and knowledge base of the faculty member concerning older adults. The rapidly growing long-term care health sector is long overdue in its wait to reap the attention of nursing students and faculty. That attention may never be fully realized without state and federal mandates to insure that there is a substantial inclusion of testing in gerontological nursing and long-term care on the national licensing examination.

NUTS AND BOLTS OF STRUCTURING CONTENT AND CLINICAL LEARNING

Widely discussed in the literature, a growing number of nurse gerontologists contend that a specific, discrete course should be taught as a required part of the nursing curriculum. Hogstel (1990) makes the point by asking why we continue to require specific courses in pediatric nursing and not in gerontological nursing? The nature of theoretical and clinical structuring in gerontological nursing is blurred by the lack of a tradition which routinely includes gerontological nursing in the curriculum. The shaping of gerontological nursing theory is still so new. The superb book by Waters, *Teaching Gerontology* (1991) is rich with numerous specific examples of teaching and learning and pithy thought provoking reasons for additional clinical concentration in the nursing facility.

The Elective

A number of surveys found that many programs choose to address gerontological nursing through an elective course. Besides the reality that only a few students will benefit from an elective, there are other inherent problems with this approach. Frequently, the elective is geared to social gerontology and not gerontological nursing in order to attract students from other disciplines. When most of the gerontological content is offered through an elective, the need for enrollees from across campus is paramount. Nursing students often view the elective with a lack of interest and limited enrollment.

Required Course

A separate required course will insure that the uniqueness of gerontological nursing content and clinical is taught. At the same time, however, specific content must also be integrated in appropriate courses throughout the curriculum. A course could be structured using the focus of chronicity and the long-term care continuum. This would provide for integration of content from a number of discrete areas as well as across the life span. Although all age groups are included, the primary focus would be on gerontological nursing content and clinical.

Whether the inclusion of gerontological nursing theoretical content is organized in an *integrated or blocked* fashion depends to a large degree on how a particular nursing school's curriculum is organized and the commitment of the school's faculty and administration. Maddox and O'Hare (1991) used a continuum of care model, where numerous health environments were used. One of the advantages of this model was the integration of gerontological nursing over the four years of college. Students had more time to assimilate knowledge and skills than is found in the typical upper division baccalaureate program. Caution is urged where only integration is used; without ongoing careful tracking, monitoring, and evaluation of content, the "integration" can be duplicative or inadequate. Spier and Yurick's (1989) students are first exposed to the healthy older adult, followed by subsequent courses in the care of acute and chronically ill older clients. The initial student experience takes place in a wellness center.

Geropsychiatry

Content and clinical can be integrated in a separate mental health nursing course or in a long-term care nursing course. Geropsychiatric clinical experience can be found in a number of long-term care settings, including adult day care, nursing facilities, and mental institutions.

Community Health

Community health nursing also fits nicely into a long-term care course. For the gerontological nursing component, initially, students should be exposed to the community dwelling elderly. Students can learn comprehensive health and functional assessments in settings such as multiple dwelling housing, senior centers, adult day care, and/or primary health care. Students would then move progressively to care for clients in the home as is found in home health nursing. Lastly, students would rotate to caring for the ill older person as is predominantly found in nursing facilities. This latter setting provides the student with an excellent opportunity to assess subtle differences in depression, dementia, and less frequently, delirium (Carignan, 1991). Students learn that interventions are different for the person who has a thought disorder and the person who has a cognitive impairing process. Regardless of the setting, health promotion should be emphasized.

Clinical Sites

Elderly housing is an excellent site to establish clinical contacts. Federally funded housing, congregate housing, and domiciliaries usually welcome the opportunity to have student nurses on the premises. Another possibility is the Continuing Care Retirement Community (CCRC). Here students can see the benefits of having a continuum of social and health services as a vital component in assisting elders to remain independent as long as possible. Students observe that functioning is influenced by the environment, where health status and longevity are facilitated by the ability to support activities of daily living, safety, and security (Carp, 1977). Because the quality of care found in CCRCs varies, faculty may wish to determine if the CCRC has been accredited. Additionally, faculty may find that the community dwelling portion of the CCRC is superior to the nursing facility setting of the CCRC (or conversely).

There has been substantial discussion on the placement of the nursing facility experience. Surveys find that the nursing facility clinical experience is offered early in the nursing curriculum. Tollett and Thornby (1982) found that a majority of graduate nurse respondents did not agree that the nursing home experience was appropriate as an initial experience. Bahr (1990) believes that initial skill learning at a nursing facility may be at the expense of preparing nurses who will shun a potential career in gerontological nursing. She feels that such a curriculum design would be ethically compromised. Tagliareni (1991) makes the case that the more seasoned advanced student will be able to deal with the complexities of the frail older adult. The senior student brings a level of skill attainment and knowledge base that will assist in assessing and promoting a restorative nursing focus and that promotes maintenance of function. *The rationale for the later timing of this clinical experience enables faculty to stress issues such as funding politics, quality of care, and complexity of clients who have multifactorial diseases.*

Hospital-Based Long-Term Care

Many acute care settings now have skilled nursing units that focus on restorative and rehabilitative nursing care of the older adult. Often, these settings have higher registered nurses to patient ratio, which promotes the use of the nurse's ability to individualize care plans (Mahoney, 1991). Acute care usually has a higher proportion of professional and advanced degree nurses whose responsibilities take them to the long-term care units; these professionals can be role models available for student learning.

Special Care Units

The nursing home that has a special care unit (SCU) will provide a wider variety of assignments for student clinicals. Studies estimate that between 11–25 percent of people with AIDS currently need long-term care; they would be placed on the SCU. The resident who has AIDS offers students and faculty a wider range of discussion topics and experiences previously not seen in the older resident group. For example, typically the course of dementia in most older residents is slow and insidious. When dementia occurs in the AIDS resident, it is frequently dramatic, rapid, and sporadic. Furthermore, when treatment is aggressive, it is frequently reversible. Intensity of nursing care varies with progression of the illness. Medications require close monitoring. Students can learn about family and social issues.

As SCUs become the norm, more facilities will have an Alzheimer's Unit (AU) where additional geropsychiatric experiences can be gained. The AU can provide an example of a protective environment, where maintenance of functioning prevails. Faculty have to be careful in selecting the AU for the clinical experience to assure that the AU is simply not a euphemism for 'housing' residents with behavioral problems.

Computers in the Nursing Facility

In the nursing home environment, students can have hands-on experience which is less hectic than in acute care. Computers are being used for patient classification, staff utilization reports, fiscal operations, laboratory diagnostics, care planning, the federally mandated minimum data sets, and interdisciplinary care plans. Molis (1992) feels that computers can cut documentation time by at least 50 percent, making nurses available for closer resident monitoring and hands on care.

Hurdles to Overcome

In addition to faculty stereotyping of both the aged and nursing facilities, there is a scarcity of good nursing facility models. Perhaps the greatest challenge faculty will find is that teaching in the nursing facility has to be different from traditional teaching in the acute care setting. To change students' attitude in a positive direction and to individualize restorative nursing, the medical paradigm of the acute care setting will not work. The nursing facility/home is a good setting to develop a *care oriented nursing practice*.

CONCLUSION

To summarize, regardless of where the long-term care clinical experience is obtained, of utmost importance is the careful planning and structuring of that experience. Since the older client is found in most health delivery settings, it is necessary to maximize learning for all clinical exposures. Students should be systematically exposed to increasingly complex gerontological nursing theoretical and clinical structuring, with the nursing faculty being a strategic part of that experience.

Editor's Note: The Reference Section consists of two parts. Part I contains the references for "Issues Facing Faculty in Long-Term Care." Part II contains the references for the "Nuts and Bolts" section of the paper.

REFERENCES—PART I

Bahr, Sr. R. T. (1992). *Ethical issues within the gerontological nursing curriculum.* Atlanta, GA: Southern Regional Education Board.

Bahr, Sr. R. T. (1981). Overview of gerontological nursing. In M. O. Hogstel (Ed.), *Nursing care of the older adult.* New York: John Wiley & Sons.

Bauer, A., & Roedel, R. (1992). Management of specialty units: A must for today's DON (Director of Nursing). *Provider, 18*(4), 35–38.

Bednash, G., Redman, B. K., Barhyte, D. Y., & Wulff, L. (1990). A data base for graduate education in nursing: Summary report. Washington, DC: American Association of Colleges of Nursing.

Brower, H. T. (1988). An analysis of associate degree nursing models. In *Strategies for Long-Term Care.* New York: National League for Nursing Press.

Brower, H. T. (1981). Teaching gerontological nursing in Florida. Where do we stand? *Nursing & Health Care, 11,* 543–547.

Carignan, A. M. (1992). Community college-nursing home partnership: Impact on nursing care. *Geriatric Nursing, 13*(3), 139–141.

Dye, C., & Sassenrath, D. (1979). Identification of normal aging and disease-related processes of health care professionals. *Journal of the American Geriatrics Society, 2,* 472–475, 1979.

Edel, M. K. (1986). Recognize gerontological content. *Journal of Gerontological Nursing, 12*(10), 28–32.

Gillick, M. R. (1989). Long-term care options for the frail elderly. *The Journal of the American Geriatrics Society, 37,* 198–203.

Hanson, H. A., & Waters, V. (1991). The sequence of curriculum change in gerontology. *Nursing & Health Care, 12,* 516–519.

Kane, R. L. (1991). Rethinking long-term care. *Journal of the American Geriatric Society, 38,* 704–9.

Malliarakis, D. R., & Heine, C. (1990). Is gerontological nursing included in baccalaureate nursing programs? *Journal of Gerontological Nursing, 16*(6), 4–7.

Rankin, N., and Burggrat, V. (1983). Aging in the 80's. *Journal of Gerontological Nursing, 9,* 270–275.

Rayfield, S. (1990). *Analysis of the NCLEX-RN test plan for the national council licensure examination for registered nurses.* Shreveport, LA: Sylvia Rayfield, Inc.

Robb, S., & Malinzak, M. (1981). Knowledge levels of personnel in gerontological nursing. *Journal of Gerontological Nursing, 7,* 153–158.

Taylor, Sr. C., & Gallagher, L. L. (1988). Structured learning for geriatric content. *Geriatric Nursing, 9,* 43–47.

Sullivan, K. W. (1984). *The importance, amount, and type of gerontological nursing content recommended for future bachelor of science in nursing curricula: A survey of the opinions of BSN faculty and practicing BSN graduates.* Unpublished doctoral dissertation, Manhattan, KS: Kansas State University.

Tobiason, S., Knudsen, F., Stengel, J., & Giss, M. Positive attitudes toward elderly patients. *Nursing & Health Care, 5,* 18–23.

U.S. Senate Special Committee on Aging, Federal Council on Aging and the U.S. Administration on Aging. (1988). *Aging America trends and projections.* Washington, DC: U.S. Department of Health and Human Services.

Verderer, D. N., & Kick, E. (1990). Gerontological curriculum in schools of nursing. *Journal of Nursing Education, 29,* 355–361.

Wells, T. J. (1980). *Problems in geriatric nursing care.* New York: Churchill Livingstone.

Yurchuck, R., & Brower, H. T. (1991). *Gerontological nursing curriculum issues: A regional profile.* Atlanta, GA: Southern Regional Education Board.

REFERENCES—PART II

Bahr, Sr. R. T. (1990). *Ethical issues within the gerontological nursing curriculum.* Atlanta, GA: Southern Regional Education Board.

Brower, H. T., Kolanowski, A. M., Tappen, R. M., & Dunham, R. (1984/85). Integration or separation for gerontological nursing. *Gerontology and Geriatrics Education, 5*(2), 45–53.

Brower, H. T. (1990). *Preparing future gerontological nurses: Essential content for nursing programs.* Paper presented at the educational conference of the National Gerontological Nursing Association, Washington, DC.

Burnside, I. M. (1992). *Incorporating health promotion for older adults into nursing curricula.* Atlanta, GA: Southern Regional Education Board.

Carignan, A. M. (1991). The content domain. In V. Waters (Ed.), *Teaching gerontology* (pp. 35–54). New York: National League for Nursing Press.

Carp, F. M. (1977). Impact of improved living environment on health and life expectancy, *The Gerontologist, 23*, 242–249.

Davis, B. (1980). Undergraduate education in gerontological nursing: Integration or separation. *Journal of Gerontological Nursing, 6*, 435–6.

Edel, M. K. (1986). Recognize gerontological content. *Journal of Gerontological Nursing, 12*(10), 28–32.

German, P. S., Rovner, B. W., Burton, L. C., Brant, L. J., & Clark, R. (1992). The role of mental morbidity in the nursing home experience. *The Gerontologist, 32*, 152–158.

Hogstel, M. (1990). Action is needed now. *Journal of Gerontological Nursing, 16*(6), 3.

Lee, J. L., & Cody, M. (1987). Gerontology education: In search of a core curriculum. *Journal of Gerontological Nursing, 13*(7), 13–17.

Maddox, M. A., & O'Hare, P. A. (1991). Designing clinical curriculum to foster positive student attitudes. *Journal of Gerontological Nursing, 17*(6), 29–33.

Mahoney, C. (1991). Return to independence. Lessons from a hospital long-term care unit. *American Journal of Nursing, 91*(3), 44–48.

Mason, K. (1992). Caring for people with AIDS. *Provider, 18*(5), 30–44.

Molis, D. B. (1992). Coming of age with technology. *Provider, 18*(3), 16–28.

National League for Nursing. (1988). *Strategies for Long-Term Care.* New York, NY: National League for Nursing Press.

Nelson, M. K. (1992). Gerontological nursing in the baccalaureate curriculum. *Geriatric Nursing, 18*(7), 26–30.

Smyer, M., Cohn, M., & Brannon, D. (1988). *Mental health consultation in nursing homes.* New York: New York University Press.

Solon, J. A., Kilpatrick, N. S., & Hill, M. S. (1988). Aging-related education: A national survey. *Journal of Gerontological Nursing, 14*(9), 21–26.

Spier, B. E., & Yurick, A. G. (1989). A curriculum design to influence positive student behaviors toward the elderly. *Nursing & Health Care, 10*, 265–268.

Staff. (1992). Nursing home chains incorporate AIDS care. *McKnight's LTC, 13*(3), 1, 25.

Tagliareni, E. (1991). What and how of student learning activities. In V. Waters (Ed.), *Teaching gerontology,* (pp. 65–91). New York: National League for Nursing Press.

Tappen, R. M., & Brower, H. T. (1985). Integrating gerontology into the nursing curriculum: Process and content. *Journal of Nursing Education, 24*(2), 80–82.

Tollett, S. M., & Thornby, J. (1982). Geriatric and gerontology curriculum trends. *Journal of Nursing Education, 21*(6), 16–23.

Waters, V. (Ed.). (1991). *Teaching gerontology.* New York: National League for Nursing Press.

Yurchuck, R., & Brower, H. T. (1991). *Gerontological nursing curriculum issues: A regional profile.* Atlanta, GA: Southern Regional Education Board.

4

Response to: "Issues Facing Faculty in Long-Term Care"

Sister Rose Therese Bahr

I am honored to be in the position of reactor to the excellent paper on the state of the art in gerontological nursing, education, and research presented by H. Terri Brower, who is my friend, professional colleague, and fellow champion of the cause. She, in her usual style, has provided an insightful overview of the major issues facing the profession of nursing in its awesome responsibility for preparing nurses to care for the ever-increasing number of older adults in America. I do not intend to comment on all the issues raised by Dr. Brower but will concentrate on several issues that to me are critical for the future of gerontological nursing so that the needs of the aging population in America are met in a satisfactory manner.

The issues to which I am reacting center primarily on faculty preparation, school administrators, i.e., deans and department chairs, and testing for competencies in gerontological nursing in the national nursing examination. These issues, in my opinion, address the major concerns that merit immediate attention if schools of nursing are to meet the demand so evident in the service sector for qualified gerontological nurses who are needed to care professionally for the old-old, frail, and young-old population in community and institutional settings.

Faculty

Many opportunities through workshops, institutes, and short-term course work have been offered to promote interest in gerontological nursing among faculty in schools of nursing. The attendance, for the most part, has been minimal. Even for those who attend, the message to incorporate gerontological nursing goes unheeded when it comes to the time for presenting curricular changes in nursing programs. There is a major problem in the nursing profession that after so many years, since the early 70s, (almost twenty years) the profession of nursing still remains so distant from the needs of the people it has a mandate to serve. Florence Nightingale in her early writings indicated that nursing remains viable only if it has a mandate from society. My question is: "Why are we not heeding the mandate that the aging population of our society requests of us?" What's wrong? Despite the amount of money made available for post-doctoral study, few faculty are taking advantage of the opportunity to upgrade their knowledge of aging and gerontological nursing. I would hazard a guess that the attitude problems of students not wishing to choose gerontological nursing as a career starts with the faculty who also have an attitude problem. To be based in reality means that all of us are on the continuum of aging. All persons will get old unless a traumatic event occurs that ends life much earlier. What are faculty afraid of that they shy away from content and clinical experience that evolves around care of the aged?

As noted by Dr. Brower, creative approaches have been made to assist faculty in obtaining knowledge and skill in gerontological nursing, e.g., SREB (Southern Regional Educational Board) Faculty Preparation Project. Yet, the problem of insufficient content and clinical experience remains a major concern. This NLN forum provides an opportunity to identify creative approaches and solutions to this problem. What are the steps that need to be taken to create an adequate supply of gerontological nursing faculty in the next five to ten years?

One final comment relates to a point made by Dr. Brower that "BSN programs devote so much time to community health nursing, leadership, and management that it may be more difficult for BSN educators to identify the urgency of adding more gerontological nursing content." I wish, as a former Community Health Nursing instructor, that I could agree about the "so much community health." It is a major struggle to acquire adequate credit allocation to prepare nurses to become competent in the areas of health promotion, health maintenance, and disease prevention since the major block of time in content and clinical experience in the curriculum goes to acute care nursing. A real challenge faces us in bringing reality into the nursing program curriculum such that it follows the trends of health care in America.

Administrators of Schools of Nursing

Faculty are the employees of schools of nursing administered by deans and department chairs. As noted by Dr. Brower, these administrators shape the philosophy and mission of the programs in nursing that they administer. What barriers are deans and department chairs facing in their institutions that prevent them from placing within the curriculum the necessary courses in gerontological nursing that would make the program more responsive to the needs of society? It is not possible to believe that top administrators of colleges and universities, e.g., university presidents, are interfering in curriculum development within the schools of nursing. It seems that the major responsibility for administration of the schools of nursing and the type of programs to be initiated rests with the nursing administrators and their faculties. Why the apathy? Why the malaise? Why the "dragging of feet" when it comes to the motivation needed by this group to exercise leadership in meeting needs so well demonstrated by society? It concerns me greatly that schools of nursing are willing to submit grant proposals for programs where money has been allocated for specific programs, like gerontological nursing, but once the grant monies are no longer available, the programs are terminated. Is that responsible management of programs or use of federal dollars? It seems that the principle of social justice can be evoked in such cases. Yet, that phenomenon is occurring throughout the nation. Because of this activity, and the few students that have been recruited into the gerontological nursing programs, federal monies for such programs are no longer being allocated since little results have been realized. *My question for this forum is: What actions need to be taken with deans and department chairs in schools of nursing to ensure that every nursing program has sufficient content and clinical experience in gerontological nursing to meet the societal demand of care to older adults?*

Testing for Gerontological Nursing
Competency at the National Level

In schools of nursing the driving force for curriculum development by the faculty, as noted by Dr. Brower, is NCLEX. The NCLEX test items cover a sampling of content and clinical judgment, in the major areas of nursing, needed to demonstrate safety in nursing practice. Unfortunately, the area of gerontological nursing is not represented as a specialty area in its own right. Several years ago, I did a study of the Review Study Guide which BSN, ADN, and diploma nursing students use in preparing to sit for the NCLEX examination. At that time (1991), all the examples of older adults presented an aged man or woman with acute illnesses. The options for nursing interventions related to medical-surgical nursing, not to age-specific options based on research and the knowledge base for gerontological nursing. In visiting with officials from Psychological Testing, the firm that prepares the NCLEX test items, the thrust of the examination is based on job descriptions for nursing personnel presently employed in long-term care facilities. These job descriptions represent state-of-the-art nursing care. The fallacy of this assumption is that very few nursing personnel in long-term care facilities have any formal education in the speciality of gerontological nursing. Consequently, the items on the national examination (i.e., NCLEX) as it relates to gerontological nursing contain information that is neither current practice nor state-of-the-art. This dilemma occurs every time the new examination is prepared for use in the national testing sites. The issue raised here is how to upgrade nursing care with qualified nurses who are prepared in gerontological nursing so that the job descriptions reflect current practice and thinking. This round robin approach to gerontological nursing items keeps the career options limited simply because the items themselves do not reflect accurate information nor critical thinking relative to the unique health care needs of the older population in community settings as well as in the institutional settings.

The competencies for the BSN and Master's prepared nurse in gerontological nursing were identified by a panel of nurse gerontologists at a conference hosted by the School of Nursing of Georgetown University in 1991. These competencies have been published by the National League for Nursing and could serve as the format for test item construction for NCLEX. No excuse remains for not including age-specific content and clinical examples for graduates of all programs. Let us exert pressure on the testing agencies so that such inclusion will take place in the near future.

Conclusion

The issues raised in Dr. Brower's paper and my reaction to selected issues are critical in moving this agenda off the paper and into reality, a reality that must be met within the next thirty years. As partners together, movement will be initiated through the cooperation of the National League for Nursing, will become visible, and will be seen as an invitation to all our colleagues to join us in this initiative. The ultimate winners are the aged persons who look to us for the quality of health care they need so that they can live meaningful and fulfilling lives for their remaining years. Again I ask: What are our next steps?

5

Educational Advancement for Quality in Long-Term Care

Patricia Moccia

An expected approach to a paper such as this would be for me to begin with one or all of the following:

1. The educational profile of the current supply of licensed and unlicensed personnel in long-term care. (This would be a relatively quick and, once the categories were defined, relatively non-arguable point from which to begin.)

2. One model or another of the projected demand in long-term care, in numbers and kind, of licensed and unlicensed personnel. (This could de-rail discussion as we would first need to debate the merits and restrictions of whatever model or models I presented. Not to mention, the tangents of whether to address the need or the demand, for today or the year 2010, leaving the one not chosen to fall into logical place behind the one favored.)

3. One position or another on whether our most appropriate policy and wisest investment would be for more LPNs, more associate or baccalaureate degree graduates, or more advanced practitioners. Or, I could really draw the line for debate by presenting precise numbers of a preferred skills mix, including assistive personnel. (I am certain I don't need to remind or caution us on

43

how such a discussion would keep us from the substantive, albeit non-academic, issues of delivering care.)

Instead, I have chosen to approach the topic by presenting three sets of statements developed to have us approach the challenges in long-term care as opportunities for the significant changes necessary in nursing education in general. Rather than solving only the presenting problems for long-term care, any such attempts might be developed in the broader context of the educational reform that is necessary to both: 1) operationalize Nursing's Agenda for Health Care Reform and 2) position higher education as part of the solution for the national and state budget deficits rather than part of the problem.

Set One re-frames the discussion to focus not solely on the educational advancement of one individual or even an aggregate of individuals but rather on long-term care as much a vital part of the educational sector as the delivery side. Set Two reconceptualizes the system itself and each of the system's components including direct care providers, patients, faculty, students, and others. Set Three revisits the ethical questions posed by Collopy, Boyle, and Jennings on the moral ecology of long-term care.

SET ONE—LTC AS A LABORATORY
FOR THE SCHOLARSHIP OF APPLICATION

1. Long-term care services cannot be separate from a comprehensive non-institution centered health care system.

2. Long-term care institutions can be developed as nursing centers with diversified community services.

3. Long-term care institutions can be used as the hub for all student clinical experiences.

4. Such experiences can be modelled so as to break past boundaries between education and service, theory and practice, and educational programs.

SET TWO—LTC AND ITS
COMPONENTS RECONCEPTUALIZED

1. Nursing homes as communities.
2. Communities connected through technology.
3. Residents as active contributors to the larger community, e.g., radio programs, seniors therapeutic touch programs, tutors, foster grandparents, etc.
4. Providers as students; students as providers; both as research assistants.
5. Faculty as anthropologists.

SET THREE—THE MORAL ECOLOGY OF LTC

1. Ethics of community
2. Residents as Moral Agents
3. Family and Staff as Moral Agents

Discussion   Having seen my approach, you can see what I am not about. Earlier in this conference, we started with certain assumptions which apply to this discussion, namely, that all of the personnel who are currently working in long-term care services, wherever they are, need increased education for advancement. It does not matter what category of worker we are talking about—nursing assistant, diploma graduate, associate degree, baccalaureate, masters—even the nurse who has certification in gerontology as advanced practice—education is needed because long-term care has changed dramatically in the last few years from what we knew it to be.

Be assured, also, that this is consistent with the challenges facing our faculty in other specialties. Whatever specialty people were prepared for has changed dramatically because of changes in two significant systems. Both the delivery system and the educational systems, as we know them, are developed to reinforce, reproduce, extend, and diversify certain relationships between people and their community. Delivery has changed dramatically and education is being asked to take on those changes also.

I ask us to think, therefore, that the current systems—both delivery, which we have spent a considerable amount of time on—but even more, education, do not serve the new order. These two systems do not serve the new relationships that we need to think about when we're talking about long-term care. In reviewing the papers that have been published over the last several years, I suggest we follow-up on what was said earlier in this conference: that long-term care should be conceptualized as a series of relationships—a series of relationships that forms a certain community—a community that is not local in place, but in fact extends extra-site, cross-sites, and uses the technology that allows us to be national and global.

As an educator, and from that perspective, I would tell people in the industry that we are looking for a place to bring our students where they can learn certain things. We are looking for a place to put into practice some of the theories and philosophies that we have been talking about for the past several years: talking about preparing students for community-based services—talking about preparing students for new relationships with communities, families, and significant others. We are looking for a place, in fact, where we can prepare our students to learn. If we are talking about educating for sustaining relationships over time within a context of community (as Sr. Donley described in her definition of quality), then I think that we as educators are looking for a spot where students can come and learn the range of things that they can no longer learn in either academia or the more traditional sites.

There has been a pendulum swing in nursing education—from practice-based education to theory-based education—and now, in reaction to that, the pendulum swings back to a practice focus of education. But it is a new practice setting. And it is a practice setting where there are new power relationships.

What we are looking for is a different social institution within the community that can serve multiple pieces and populations. The diversified long-term care service setting might be that place where we can bring our students. If we bring our students there, and develop nursing centers where traditional long-term care services are delivered, then we can have a nursing education experience that will prepare students for the multiple possibilities of employment opportunities they will have after graduation.

A nursing center where long-term care services are delivered is, in its broadest sense, also an employer of the community. As we know, hospitals, and to some degree, long-term care institutions, are the major points of entry into the work force for many people. The nursing center has been conceptualized as a *learning organization*. It is also a laboratory of nursing scholarship; the faculty is an employee of the nursing center, not the long-term care service nor the educational system. I think that the idea of faculty in relationship to different kinds of institutions is one that we need to look at as we talk about changing relationships.

If we had a nursing center where long-term care services were diversified and if it conceptualized itself in terms of its many responsibilities—employer of the community, deliverer of services, a laboratory for scholarship—we could then fulfill one of the most basic principles of education. We could begin to think of *learning teams* that include nursing assistants, LPNs, ADNs, BSNs, the administrators, and the traditional faculty. This group, this learning team, rather than a dichotomy between provider and faculty, are in fact one of several learning teams within a learning organization.

In this newly conceptualized nursing center, everybody learns a little, everybody delivers a little; AD, baccalaureate, and master's faculty are now also delivering services. Assistant personnel are receiving academic credit for practice; they are validating their technologic expertise. AD people are receiving baccalaureate credit; LPNs are receiving AD credit. The point is that the whole educational enterprise is ripped from its usual moorings of the educational 'institution' and put back into practice—and is owned by the learning team that included both administrators and faculty.

As you read in the statements developed to approach challenges in long-term care, I alluded to faculty as anthropologists. The learning team could take responsibility for two, three years, and follow a patient through their lived experience. That person's accessing different parts of the spectrum of health care services could be something for the entire team to learn about. In short, we have to help faculty break out of their boxes, whatever the box, whether it be the medical model box, or the setting box, whatever. Bring back the faculty, re-socialize them, re-skill them (whatever the least insulting term is) to be the much more coordinated, collaborative, non-specialist, generalist educator of helping people look at patterns and follow an individual's living experience.

6

Response to: "Educational Advancement for Quality in Long-Term Care"

Clair Martin

It is clear that Pat Moccia is telling us that we have the opportunity, at this point in political, social, and health 'time,' to look at things in a dramatically different way. The usual and customary way of 'doing' nursing education is not functional; we have heard this repeatedly. The old paradigm of nursing education is already dead. What we do know is that we have a huge stack of unsolved (and unsolvable?) problems in nursing education—with the usual and customary way of doing things. As educators, we cannot pretend to be significant players in health care reform without nursing education reform. And that does not mean tinkering around the edges. What Moccia has presented is a completely different context for 'doing' nursing education; and I like it. To make her ideas more explicit, she has stated that there is no longer a separate culture for nursing education and a separate culture for practice. If nursing intends to be a significant player in health care reform, we must have a *culture for nursing*. It appears inevitable that nursing education will have to relinquish some of those wonderful, safe relationships and practices to which we persistently adhere. Perhaps, creating an entirely new environment for providing care, i.e., the nursing center, is the vehicle which will enable us to do that.

At Emery, we began several community-based nurse managed care centers. One was in a low-income housing unit and another was in a middle class senior community. We assessed the unmet needs in both communities. It was surprising to find that there was no difference in the unmet health needs between the two communities. By the time I left that area, faculty and students were asking to have part of their learning opportunities in these long-term care or elderly facilities, simply because it was different. We were not asking them to 'do' gerontology in the same way that we had required them to perform gerontological nursing. They were participating in an experiment where the knowledge and skill of nursing was used to facilitate people's ability independently with managed care.

In the nursing centers/learning organizations described by Moccia, there appeared to be a great value and reliance on accommodation and cooperation. In nursing, we have always put a premium on those two characteristics. But I think that the environment of the care center envisioned by Moccia relies much more strongly on expertise in collaboration and competition. You have to bring to the table fairly equal resources in order to collaborate or compete. Indeed, your competitor at one moment may be your collaborator at another. While nursing education has done some work on developing assertiveness skills in our graduates, it would appear that we need to inculcate or teach the concepts Moccia alluded to, e.g., cooperation. The learning team partnership of students, practitioners, and faculty must be based on the notion of *collaboration among equals.* This means shared decision making among persons with equal— but different—resources to bring to the table. There is no question that the *student as partner* is a foreign concept. There would be problems and a failure of nerve when unspoken sets of expectations (between student and faculty, each for the other) get in the way of the kind of risk-taking that Pat Moccia's proposal requires.

Another factor to think about in this 'new community' is the fact that newcomers to America who are entering the work force are not only from diverse cultures and educational backgrounds, but one in four will be women. It is estimated that these women are going to spend more of their time caring for their parents than they did for their children. So, when we plan this new community, we need to understand that the players may be significantly different from what they are at the present time.

Education is in crisis at all levels. One of the issues we have not talked about is the excuse promulgated by the schools of nursing that they are not doing what needs to be done (e.g., curriculum reform) because "the raw material that is coming isn't what it used to be." We need, there-fore, to engage ourselves in the political arena to insure that education is a total process from beginning to end. In emphasizing the investment in developing human capital, it seems that in long-term care we are still very much committed to the old idea that we have an inexhaustible supply of human resources. We complain about not having enough people, but the way we behave we use them up, discard them, and replace them. We need to advance our provider's knowledge and skill abilities, not just to be sure that the care meets a higher level of excellence but because (some of) the basic human needs of that worker, that individual, need to be met through satisfaction with work, through feedback. It is not just salary. The kind of human dignity that makes a committed worker and member of a group comes through an increase in knowledge and productivity.

Faculty and deans are not malevolent individuals. The problem is that our usual and customary methods are not working, but they are the only ones we know. So, people get burned out by working harder and harder at what is working less and less. Moccia's model intrigues me.

7

Education Articulation Models and the Nursing Home Industry

Paul Willging

Editor's Note: The paper by Ellen Tishman was written for the conference in order to give participants a sense of the context of long-term care relative to educational needs and access. It was expected that the participants would have read its contents before the Willging presentation.

EDUCATION ARTICULATION AND THE LONG-TERM CARE FIELD

Ellen Tishman

This paper is intended to provide background for discussion about educational needs and articulation. It begins with a description of professional (i.e., RN) shortages and other staffing issues. The pressures and challenges of the nursing shortage are exacerbated in long-term care facilities. Up to 34 percent of nursing homes report "severe" RN shortages; the vacancy rate exceeds 20 percent as compared to a 7–8 percent vacancy rate in acute care. Vacancy rates of licensed practical nurses (LPNs) and certified nursing assistants (CNA) are higher. The Secretary's Commission on Nursing estimates that 21,000–26,000 more RNs are needed to staff

53

nursing homes (1988, p. 11). Obviously, this does not reflect the need for LPNs or CNAs.

Only 8 percent of all working RNs are employed by long-term care institutions. Bedside care is most often provided by the assistants and LPNs. Nursing staffing, therefore, is heavily skewed toward these providers of care. The typical nursing home, in 1985, employed an average of 31 nursing assistants (i.e., aides and orderlies), seven LPNs, and five RNs per 100 beds. Despite the fact that registered nurse employment in the nursing home sector increased by 22 percent from 1981 to 1986, the Secretary's Commission report pointed to the real-life effects of the shortage on the patients (residents) and the staff: the substantial stress under which RNs may work raises concern about the quality of patient care; *the increased workload alters the way RNs care for their patients.* The ramifications of the problem are troubling: poor quality care; media and congressional exposés and scandals; more heavy-handed government/ regulatory action; more ("patient neglect and abuse") litigation against providers and professionals; lack of access to long-term care; unwillingness of existing staff to work under these conditions; and *poor clinical practice settings for nursing and other health care students.*

To think about providing education articulation models for the nursing home field, it is necessary to know the number of different nursing staff populations and their maximum level of education. Seventy percent of the nursing department staffing is non-licensed, i.e., nurse assistants (CNAs). Of the remaining licensed group, 17–20 percent are LPNs. As of 1985, more than 56 percent of the RNs are diploma school graduates. This has probably shifted slightly to reflect an influx of ADN graduates to nursing home employment. Relatively recent statistics indicate that only 6 percent of the directors of nursing in long-term care have a master's degree (in advanced clinical practice, management, business, etc.). There is ample evidence that the baccalaureate nurse is not attracted to long-term care, for a variety of reasons. The nursing home is heavily reliant, therefore, on the licensed practical nurse. The "seasoned" LPNs tend to be well-prepared to work not only with the bedside care needs of the residents but with the day-to-day running of a nursing unit; the industry is in their debt.

It should not be surprising, then, that the long-term care providers are concerned about efforts to limit educational programs for LPNs and to limit their ability to practice. In AHCAs (American Health Care

Association) view, there is a role in nursing homes for nurses from a variety of educational backgrounds. The 'ideal' nursing team to meet the complex needs of today's nursing home resident, should include LPNs, nurses from diploma, ADN and BSN programs, *and* the certified nursing assistant. Having stated this, it is unlikely that the nursing home sector will get more professional/registered nurses if diploma and LPN schools of nursing continue to close or if licensure opportunities are eliminated. It is for these reasons that AHCAs board of governors recently approved a position statement that supports four levels of entry into nursing practice: LPN, ADN, diploma, and baccalaureate. The position paper argues for support of graduate programs in nursing "specifically gerontology, which contribute to the body of theoretical, research, skill, and advanced practice in long-term care." It is only through a commitment to maintain and expand the nursing profession by provider and nursing organizations that we can reshape and expand the nursing pool—not by contracting or impeding entry or movement within the system. The integrity, i.e., quality, of long-term care services is dependent on the availability of nurses at all levels of educational preparation who are well prepared to join the ranks of LTC nursing service.

Educational Mobility

One of the potential solutions aimed at alleviating the shortage of nurses is the *development of flexible nursing education opportunities.* Coordinated systems for educational mobility, career ladders, and articulation models are pathways that facilitate upward mobility from one level of nursing education and practice to another. The education articulation system *should recognize past experience, competencies, and education* of each individual advancing through the system (Moore & Simendinger, 1989). This recognizes that effective recruitment and retention starts with the people already working in the field. Some articulation models build in the recognition of program and course content through the student's validated work experience. Some models, for nursing assistant career and educational advancement, have interim levels, such as "advanced certified nurse assistant" or a CNA "specialist" or "senior CNA."

Given the number and mix of nursing staff in the nursing home, the care that each level/classification provides is uniquely different from the roles that these practitioners provide in other settings. Research indicates that RNs in long-term care spend the majority of their time on management-related functions. The limited registered nurse time per patient day influences the work responsibilities of RNs employed by nursing homes as compared to RNs employed in hospitals. *Less than 10 percent of RNs currently employed in nursing homes deliver direct patient care.* During a usual work week, RNs in nursing homes report their primary work involvement, (i.e., in percent reporting they are always involved in the activity) as follows: assigning and supervising nursing staff (64%); observing and documenting resident care (63%); administering routine therapies such as medications and treatments (53%); determining resident care plans (47%); evaluating and modifying care plans (37%); administering complex therapies (26%); teaching and counseling residents (19.5%), (Secretary's Commission on Nursing, *Support Studies and Background Information*, Vol. II, 1988). This poses interesting caveats when analyzing the competencies that CNAs, LPNs, and RNs acquire while working in long-term care facilities and is a *critical point* if we are to recognize work experience in developing models of articulation and course credit. The argument, then, is that in addition to recognizing previous (formal) education, the education system needs to recognize work experience and nursing competencies specific to long-term care.

The question, then, is "How do the current career mobility programs and articulation plans reflect the knowledge, competencies, and skills of nurses in long-term care?" Review of the current models of educational articulation are disappointing. Most educational programs reflect current curriculum design largely rooted in the hospital/acute care model. They do not take into account the experience-based skills and competencies acquired (by the nurse) in the long-term care setting.

Career Mobility and Articulation
Models in Long-Term Care

The tradition of articulation in long-term care has been limited to isolated models and episodic implementation of coordinated systems for nursing students to move within the educational system. Generally, long-term care settings lack incentives which have been demonstrated to retain staff: a working environment that provides career development opportunities and a *reward system* that recognizes education, experience, and productivity. This makes creating mobility in this setting more pressing and, yet, more challenging. The Commission on Nursing noted that career advancement is an important factor in both recruitment and retention of nurses (in all settings) but, with few exceptions, these opportunities are limited or non-existent in long-term care settings (*Final Report*, 1991).

An array of barriers exists such that even those students who are interested in educational and career advancement confront a restrictive and inefficient process. One of the most vexing barriers to educational advancement stems from the admission and transfer policies of individual academic institutions which results in repetitious courses and clinical instruction that many registered nurse students find "wasteful of their time and money," (Institute of Medicine Report, 1983). For experienced nurses, duplicative teaching in the clinical areas is highly frustrating. Because of the unique experiences of long-term care nurses and because of the inevitable barriers, a strong case needs to be made for 1) reaching consensus on the competencies of nursing staff in long-term care, thereby defining the skills and functions of all nursing staff; 2) using these competencies as the basis for models that recognize past experience; and 3) creating change within schools of nursing and provider organizations to encourage and facilitate career advancement.

There is support for recognition of competencies in the literature. Grant (1979) stated that demonstration of competence should be independent of time served in formal educational settings. *Since the competencies in long-term care are specific to the practice setting, it is critical that educators review and accept a set of "setting-specific" competencies that are uniformly recognized by academic institutions as students move through the system (or around the country).* These models become "ideal" when students are able to overcome any knowledge deficit in a self-paced, nontraditional manner (Lethbridge et al, 1990). What becomes clear is that models based on competencies rarely conform to generic curricula. Evidence suggests, in fact, that competency-based recognition creates a need for an atypical, nonconforming curriculum. "In allowing any or all of the nursing components to be challenged, students differ radically from each other in credits earned during competence assessment. They seldom conform to the ordered nursing content in the generic curriculum. For example, it is possible for a student to successfully challenge objectives related

to alterations in oxygenation but know little about respiratory functioning in the well individual. Because of their work experience, they synthesize material differently from generic students new to nursing. . . .
Therefore, the simple-to-complex nursing curriculum used for generic students may be presented using the same principles of learning but with the
content differently ordered" (Lethbridge et al, 1990, p. 65).

We need to create a balance between traditional methods of articulation through evaluation and assessment of academic preparation with
a focus on competency-based articulation through evaluation of nursing
experience. Nursing experience is assessed through documentation of
how life and work experiences translate to educational outcomes or
competencies. Faculty assess how these experiences meet established educational objectives. The list of competencies prepared for this paper
(*See Appendix B. Ed.*) should become the basis for this 'portfolio' and
an agreed upon mechanism for recognizing long-term care nursing
experience.

Assumptions and Recommendations

Underlying premises of the recommendations are:

a. Models of articulation should be based on a reward system that
   recognizes education, experience, and productivity.
b. Past experience can be assessed through a portfolio of nursing
   experience.
c. The portfolio of nursing experience should be based on a set of
   minimum competencies. These competencies should be set nationally and revised on a state-by-state basis pursuant to specific
   Nurse Practice Acts.

Based on these assumptions, it is recommended that long-term care and
organized nursing work in partnership to create the necessary changes,
some of which were addressed in this paper. We should be held accountable for actualizing the following components:

A. To create recognition for articulation models that recognize past experience as well as educational achievement.

Step 1. Create consensus for minimum competencies.

Step 2. Use challenge tests, credit waivers, and portfolios of past experience as the basis for minimizing redundancy and repetition as students move through the nursing education system.

B. To create an environment in the nursing facility that promotes and provides career development opportunities.

Step 1. Sensitize nursing home administrators and nursing staff to career development and career advancement.

Step 2. Create alliances between nursing facilities and educational institutions *as well as* between different educational institutions preparing various levels of nurses.

Step 3. Foster opportunities for nursing facilities to become clinical practice sites for students.

Step 4. Promote incentives for working nurses to go back to school: flexibility in shifts, assignments, and responsibilities; provision of child care, transportation, tuition benefits, etc.

C. To expand nursing curricula to include a stronger geriatric component (coursework and clinical) and require a gerontological nursing component for NLN certification.

D. To promote nursing and long-term care to secondary and post-secondary students.

E. To promote the accessibility and availability of scholarships for nursing students in the articulation and generic tracks.

Conclusion

It is this author's contention that we will recruit more nurses to long-term care and enhance care-giving if nursing organizations and long-term care providers work together, state by state, at the local level as well as the national level, to create opportunities that afford exciting, rewarding, and challenging experiences. *We must clearly state in our messages to future and current long-term care nurses that providers and educators fully support, recognize, and facilitate career advancement.* We must work together to eliminate the barriers which restrict movement within the system and up the career ladder. Industry and education have the combined power to "force" providers to encourage nurse assistants and nurses to go back to school *and* to provide the support systems that facilitate their return. We certainly appear to have the combined power to influence educators to rethink the current systems which link academic institutions together and which link academic institutions to nursing facilities. We need to work together to insure that every nursing student spends time in a long-term care facility learning the challenges of long-term care nursing. I am assuming that we can work together to make sure that all schools of nursing regard care of the elderly as a critical curricular component.

COMMENTARY ON "EDUCATION ARTICULATION MODELS AND THE NURSING HOME INDUSTRY"

Paul Willging

Prefacing my comments about education articulation models, I will address two issues that are germane to our topic, quality of care mechanisms. The two issues are perceptions of the nursing home by professionals as well as the public, and the shortage of nurses in long-term care. It has been said that seldom has an Institute of Medicine (IOM) study been essentially translated, word for word, into legislation—this, in reference to the Nursing Home Reform Laws and OBRA '87. This should not be that difficult to understand; the nursing home industry was extremely supportive of the legislation. The industry, surprising as it may seem to some, can be innovative as well as forceful and risk-taking. Credit must be given, also, to the National Citizen's Coalition for Nursing Home Reform. They pulled together consensus groups and lobbying groups which dealt with almost all the major provisions that ultimately went to the legislature. That is probably the reason that there was as much parallelism in the legislation with the study. Of the hundred or so recommendations which emanated out of the IOM study, the American Health Care Association (AHCA) opposed only about four or five of them, and some of them were clearly not implementable under any circumstances. For example, an IOM recommendation which the industry opposed was that a nursing facility should not be permitted to hire a nursing assistant unless that individual had completed a course at an accredited academic institution. This was an unreasonable recommendation, one that would clearly have caused hardship on any nurse assistant. It was fairly well recognized that it was unworkable even though this recommendation would have met its major purpose, i.e., to try to get a handle on abuse of residents by nurse assistants. If that recommendation had been promulgated into regulation, there would no longer have been any resident abuse by nurse assistants because there would not have been any more nurse assistants.

I wish to suggest that the OBRA '87 legislation and regulations have been received very positively by the industry. Yes, there was some initial panic about implementation and costs, but by and large, OBRA's requirements reflected innovation that was already coming from within the nursing home industry itself. *Almost everything in OBRA '87 had been pioneered somewhere across the land,* by no means unanimously, but by many of the better nursing facilities. The industry did have *one serious problem: the issue of nursing coverage and staffing requirements in OBRA '87.* Without exception, the IOM staffing recommendation of twenty-four hour nursing coverage was supported by organized nursing. The industry made a vigorous stand and by an excruciatingly close vote in the full Commerce and Energy Committee, the RN staffing requirement was modified to one shift of RN coverage and twenty-four hours of licensed nurse coverage. (The waiver of the nursing coverage requirement had to be created in order to deal with the shortage of RNs—but it has very stringent reporting and management activities.) The nursing home industry's battle against the twenty-four hour RN coverage should not be construed as proof that the industry is unable to recognize the close correlation between quality care and professional nursing coverage. In truth, the absence of RN staff is one of our biggest problems in terms of achieving the kind of quality levels we want.

The problem, then, is not a failure of the industry to recognize the correlation between quality and professional staffing. Rather, it is a recognition of the market realities, recruitment and retention issues, and, that such a provision in regulation would come back to haunt us and imperil reasonable operations (through penalties, deficiencies, etc.). The current registered nurse vacancy rate in nursing homes is twenty percent; this is

much higher than acute care or any other nurse practice setting. What
is it in the environment that nourishes this continuing vacancy/shortage
problem? Nurses perceptions of nursing homes, of working in a nursing
home, reflects the public's general perception. A recent public opinion research poll (done by AHCA) was unsurprising, and we were not too
thrilled with what was found. While the nursing home industry does not
rank at the bottom of the barrel, we are viewed with the same pejorative
connotations as government, insurance agents, and used car salespersons.
One unexpected and dismaying finding was that individuals who had had
some experience with nursing homes, e.g., those with a family member as
a resident, had the same unfavorable regard for nursing homes as did individuals with no experience of the care and the environment. This splash
of cold water has given the industry some sense of the direction it needs to
take over the next several years.

Perception of the nursing home setting remains one of our greatest
problems. *Our other major problem is that support for nursing in the nursing
home is virtually non-existent.* The nursing home domain of practice is not
a laid back environment. There is very little in the way of support personnel to help nurses do their job. Nurse-to-patient ratios are drastically different between the nursing home setting and acute care. According to
the Secretary's Commission on Nursing report, there are ninety-eight
RNs for every one hundred hospital beds/patients. In a one-hundred bed
nursing facility, there are 5.2 RNs. Nurses have to perform functions and
tasks in nursing homes which they do not have to do in most other health
care centers. Nursing home nursing is a tough job and we don't pay them
anything for that tough job. The data is clear on compensation: there is
approximately a thirty percent differential between salaries paid to all
nursing personnel (not just RNs) in nursing homes in comparison to
nursing personnel in acute care. The problems then are two fold: a public
perception of nursing homes that is not flattering and a rate of pay for a
tough job that is only seventy percent of the going rate. Recruitment
problems crystallize when confronted with this kind of information.

The demographics of the aging population should convince us that
there will be an increasing need for nursing facility services, particularly
for persons over the age of 85 years, i.e., the old-old. Twenty-two percent
of all Americans over the age of eighty-five years are in nursing homes.
And while the United States population as a whole is going to grow by
approximately twenty-five to thirty percent over the next thirty years, the

population of the old-old is expected to grow by four hundred percent. Unless we have a change in utilization factors, there is going to be a staggering need and demand for facilities, resources, and obviously, for nursing personnel. Data from an Urban Institute study which looked at a huge range of variables with respect to the need for institutional care predicts that by the year 2010 there will be a need for 3 million nursing home beds. This is twice the number of beds that is currently available; this is a prediction that says that the number of beds needed must double in eighteen years. In addition to asking the import of these data on the need for nursing personnel, we must look at acuity levels, also. Twenty-five years ago, the average Activities of Daily Living (ADL) dependency in nursing homes was that an individual was dependent in one out of four ADLs. Today, the average ADL dependency of residents in nursing homes is four out of five. Sixty percent of the residents have some form of senile dementia, usually Alzheimer's type. The resident is also sicker, clinically sicker. This situation will become exacerbated because the ratio of nursing home beds to the elderly is at its lowest point in the past ten to fifteen years. Why? States are refusing to allow construction and banks are refusing to provide financing. *In an attempt to respond to the decline in resources, i.e., beds and access, nursing homes are admitting sicker and sicker patients (residents).* Sixty percent of the Medicaid dollar currently goes for institutional care. This explains why you are seeing a 'new' type of resident in the nursing home and why we are hearing of, and looking for, new programs oriented toward alternative, non-institutional arrangements for care and services.

There is no question that OBRA '87 forced the industry to recognize that there are functions in nursing homes that cannot be performed by licensed practical nurses. However, there *are* functions in nursing homes which cannot be performed by anyone but a baccalaureate prepared nurse. The industry is beginning to recognize the complexity of care. The educational levels of our practitioners, on whom we have relied for so many years, are simply not keeping up with the acuity and coordinating needs for complexities of care. "Diversification" has become a buzz word in some nursing homes; that is, that since there is not much money to be made in caring for the almost ambulatory, chronic disease patient, why bother? But to many, if not most nursing homes, involvement with acute or semi-acute care of the older adult is taking hold. Nursing homes are setting up special care units (SCU), for

Alzheimer's disease, for rehab, for a whole variety of diseases and conditions. The demand for professional nursing will increase, not decrease. We are already seeing that while the ratio of beds to population is decreasing, the staffing is increasing. The demand for additional nursing personnel will grow exponentially. The bottom line, then, is that the industry has to "home-grow" our own nursing personnel, our own nurses. We cannot recruit in the traditional sense of going into the market. Paradoxically, nursing homes have now become a training ground for nurse assistants who leave the nursing facility to go to work in the hospital—usually because the pay is better.

The long-term care industry needs to do a better job in identifying those people within our ranks who are either already prepared or who are ready to begin the steps up the career ladder. We need to provide the incentives and we need to provide the reimbursement, e.g., tuition coverage. For staff to enter an educational program (articulated or not), the nursing home has to be able to offer flexible hours and shifts. The industry needs to become part of the solution but to do so it will need help, obviously, from professional nursing, particularly from the schools of nursing. This is a three-sided collaboration: nursing schools, nursing organization, and the industry itself. In truth, the industry is not as sensitized to this collaborative need for survival as it needs to be. Some of the state associations are beginning to recognize the outlines of the problem as are some of the multi-facility corporations. In Oklahoma, the RN (and licensed nurse) shortage subsequent to the OBRA staffing requirement is so severe that there are hundreds of waivers (for the RN or licensed nurse requirement) in effect. But waivers do not solve the problem nor can they go on indefinitely; residents need to be taken care of in nursing homes and these residents are ill and debilitated. The nursing facility response throughout much of the state has been to identify staff who can move to higher positions of work and responsibility. They have begun to select nurse assistants (CNAs) that have the potential to become LPNs; LPNs who can become ADNs; and so on. There are some models already in operation that offer this kind of educational and career mobility, for example, the LINC Program (Ladders in Nursing Careers) in New York State.

As part of the collaboration between education and industry, there is a need to really look at the possibility that experience in lieu of the formal educational experience is a sound principle on which to develop a health care career track. This is not a new idea; there are some models doing this already. The list of minimum competencies is our (AHCAs) contribution to the dialogue, to the extant models, and to the models which are yet to be structured. The competencies reflect things which, for example, you would expect a well trained, experienced nurse assistant to know, to do. Coupled with appropriate testing programs—which should not substitute for *all* academic training but for a reasonable amount—the process of career movement could be enhanced expeditiously.

REFERENCES

Commission on the National Nursing Shortage. (1991). *Final Report, September 1991*. Washington, DC.

Grant, J. (1979). *On Competency: A Critical Analysis of Competency Evaluation*. San Francisco: Jossey-Bass Publishers.

Institute of Medicine. (1983). *Nursing and Nursing Education: Public Policies and Private Actions*. Washington, DC: National Academy Press.

Lethbridge, D. J., Tausch, J., Lynch, K. R., & Noyes, D. E. Second-step Versus Competence-based RN Baccalaureate Education in a Rural Setting. In Little, C. (1990). *Nursing & Health Care: The Supplement*. New York: National League for Nursing Press.

Marion Merrell Dow. (1992). *Managed Care Digest: Long-Term Care Edition*. Kansas City: Marion Merrell Dow, Inc.

McKibbin, R. C. (1990). *The Nursing Shortage and the 1990s: Realities and Remedies*. Kansas City: American Nurses Association.

Moore, T. F., & Simendinger, E. A. (1989). *Managing The Nursing Shortage: A Guide to Recruitment and Retention*. Rockville: Aspen Publishers, Inc.

Secretary's Commission on Nursing. (1988). *Interim Report, Volume III*. Washington, DC.

Secretary's Commission on Nursing. (1988). *Support Studies and Background Information, Volume II*. Washington, DC.

Tourigny, A. W., & Fiore, L. (1988). Nurses: Our Endangered Species. *The Journal of Long-Term Care Administration, Winter*, 19–21.

U.S. Department of Health and Human Services, Public Health Service, (1985). *The National Nursing Home Survey, 13*(97). Hyattsville: Department of Health and Human Services.

8

Response to: "Education Articulation Models and the Nursing Home Industry"

Mary Ousley

It is incumbent upon me to point out that the nursing home industry was most unhappy with the enforcement provisions that came with the OBRA '87 regulations, i.e., the revised quality assurance survey process. The approach to keeping nursing homes in compliance with OBRA '87 regulations and requirements was punitive. This is an approach that appears to work well but does not. It is counterproductive in terms of professionalism and fails to speak to the real issues in health care delivery. Furthermore, the provisions appear to be implemented haphazardly, across regions and states. The punitive approach treats all "mistakes" in practice the same; this can have a negative effect on career commitment.

There was and remains an attitude problem within the nursing profession. It seems to come primarily from education and prevents an honest appreciation of what articulation models can do. Some of the attitude is based on the erroneous assumption that individuals who enter health care occupations at a lower level are probably individuals who lack the capacity to move onward and upward in career ladders, or even into management. We have not moved forward as rapidly as we need to on articulation models. We have continuing problems with recruitment, as has been stated earlier; we are still chewing up staff and then just letting them go. Long-term care is not perceived as a creative, innovative environment. OBRA '87 essentially told the industry: change yourself or you will be changed.

One perception that has changed, within the industry as well as when viewed from the outside, is that long-term care does not just 'house' the chronically ill elderly; it provides aggressive health care through health promotion, maintenance, and treatment. Elderly who would have formerly been treated in, and remained in, acute care are now being provided that care in nursing homes. Insurance companies, as a matter of fact, are very interested in the "acute care" units in nursing homes; they are comparing costs relative to outcomes. As you know, costs of care are much less in the nursing home. So, the type of care being provided in nursing homes is changing—and so is the number, mix, and quality of the competency of nursing home personnel.

The clinical competencies put together by Tishman (*See Appendix B*. Ed.) are a good beginning. They are regulatory based but also speak to aspects of educational competencies for an articulation model. There is more to competency, however, than whether the individual knocks on the door before entering the room or addresses the resident appropriately. Competency evaluation or measures need to look at all the critical competencies of interpersonal relationships; the skills and sensitivities needed to meet the needs of resident, family, and community—in the nursing home setting. The nursing home setting *is* a different setting; it takes a special individual or special skills to master the interpersonal competencies needed.

At the Hillhaven Corporation, we have decided to look more closely at how we treat our nurses. We begin with asking the question: are we hiring the right nurses? I sometimes feel that the basic criteria for employment (of an RN) is do they walk, talk, breathe, can they make it through a typical day, and are they licensed? This sounds facetious but it has been true, all too often; it has not necessarily provided us with the highest caliber of nurses. In our attempt to identify the 'best and the brightest,' we are looking at: what nurses seem to be providing the very best care? What type of management model seems to work the best? We identified forty nurses and met with each for extensive interviewing. We wanted to know: why are you better than others? How do you manage to do a good job on your unit where others seem to be failing? Based on our survey, along with additional research, our composite of the critical competencies for professional service are: interviewing skills, leadership, and most importantly, excellent clinical skills. Out of this, we have developed a baseline of competencies that any applicant for a leadership position, including that of nursing director, must have in order for the corporation to reach its goals. The next step for us has been to identify the critical competencies needed at, or for, each level of care, i.e., from acute to sub-acute to chronic care. It is important to point out that a baseline competency is not the same as the level of proficiency that the individual must have to move to another level. A component step is to provide the education and training needs for baseline and proficiency levels of mastery. One other piece of this package is the need to offer salaries commensurate with knowledge and skills; if we have a particular level of expectation of proficiency, then we must pay for it.

The traditional nurse management model is not all that functional in long-term care. It is something we need to look at as we look at education articulation. We have not been as supportive of our nursing personnel as we should be. We have placed tremendous responsibility on nurse managers but denied them the tools of management. Accordingly, Hillhaven has moved to authorizing the nurse manager's right to manage resources, and be accountable for this, i.e., the budget. We are also encouraging our nurse managers to use their accrued benefit time, to take the time off they are entitled to, to feel 'okay' that the unit will not fall apart if they take some time off or leave at the end of their shift. Autonomy and effective time management, then, is part of our plan for the growth, development, and preservation of nurse managers.

The profession has not done enough about differentiated practice. This is not something that the nursing home industry can do by itself. There is a dramatic difference between education and training for the LPN, the ADN, the BSN. One thing the industry can, and should, take on is sensitizing and educating owners and administrators to these differences in performance based on level of education.

Articles in the public media and the survey done by AHCA did indeed reveal that public perceptions of nursing homes are not flattering. However, we have found that when people have had an experience with a nursing home setting, they come away with positive feelings about the 'place.' Not uncommonly, the public feeling is that "the nursing home in my community is good, but others are not good." Clearly, we have to work on public perceptions and attitudes.

The opportunity is clearly at hand to put together the articulation models; to have a strong partnership between long-term care and nursing education. I believe that the future of health care is in long-term care. It is not impossible to visualize that the hospital of the future will be like a satellite. It will have an emergency room, an intensive care unit, a surgical unit, and a few beds. The provision of care and services once the person has passed that point is going to be in a different place. That 'different place' will be institutional long-term care, nursing centers. It is a good idea to move away from the old language of "nursing home" and call it what it is, or will be: nursing facility, nursing center, resident center.

9

Policy and Funding Implications of Programs Providing Education in Long-Term Care Institutions

Ethel L. Mitty

Editor's Note: The author of this paper was unable to be present at the invitational conference. Drawing on leads and issues noted in the Abstract, which was included in the conference papers, Sr. McNicholl introduced the topic. The complete article is printed below and is preceded by Sr. McNicholl's comments.

Sr. McNicholl: *I believe that there are two issues, with respect to educational programs in long-term care, at the outset: 1) there is an absence of programs within the institution, other than what is mandated by OBRA '87; 2) there is a dearth of nursing school programs coming to nursing homes for clinical experience. One thrust of Mitty's discussion about policy and funding implications is her assertion that educational institutions are not the sole repositories of knowledge; there should be a partnership that is established in any of these nursing institutions so that there is shared learning. Going beyond the OBRA-mandated requirements for continuing education for nursing assistants, Mitty apparently feels that there should be some mandatory pieces of continuing education for the nurses and directors of nursing in long-term care. There is a need to define "long-term care" because the kind of nursing that is needed in the setting is changing. What is the educational content and mode, indeed, what are the educational needs given the shifting functions and services of long-term institutional care? There is a need for political decisions which have funding implications. In addition to agreement on the competencies needed for long-term (i.e., gerontological nursing) practice, Mitty appears to be asking us to address faculty competency for long-term care nursing education. Faculty need to be competent in the skills aspects of nursing home care, not just the didactics. We need to address the cost-effectiveness of using geriatric nurse practitioners (GNP) in the long-term care setting. The Rand study found that there were significant savings in health systems cost and in resident well-being. What kinds of nurses do we need in the current and future institutional long-term care setting? [Conclusion of prefatory remarks]*

Initial reaction to the request to provide input on policy and funding implications of programs providing education in long-term care was "what programs?" A first response was to flip the title of the article in order to show that long-term care nursing service is not a passive, ignorant receptacle waiting for the breath of knowledge which could come only from academe. We, the leaders and spokespersons for health care education, research, policy development, and service have got to stop referring to the long-term care sector as one which needs 'things' done *to* and *for* it. There are enormous strengths and skills within long-term care; they have been unheralded, unrewarded, and untapped. An alternate title is therefore proposed: *Policy and Funding Implications for LTC Institutions as Partners and Affiliates in Educational Programs.* This new title is more appropriate, timely, and sensitive to the feelings and interests of nursing home staff. It also addresses the quest for quality of care of the elderly as surely as does the original title.

Historically, the use of the nursing home as an educational setting, i.e., a clinical campus, is not new. There has been a shift, however, in the amount of time spent at the site and when, in the course of the students' education, the experience occurs. As recently as 1983, nursing homes were used to introduce the student (notably, the ADN student) to basic nursing care, e.g., bedmaking, baths, transfer, feeding, etc. The student group generally spent one full day per week for the entire semester, on site, and with a "teacher." In some programs, specific residents were selected jointly by the faculty and the nurse in charge. Despite the additional work involved for the charge nurse, e.g., changing assignments, assuring that there was sufficient (extra) linen on hand, the nursing home staff appeared to enjoy their role as teachers. This pleasure was also frequently expressed by the nurse assistants; (we do not believe it had anything to do with their having a lighter case load that day). This scenario changed as the nursing education curriculum changed. Student nurses were not coming for the "basics" but for the 'psychosocial' component of their education. Students were assigned one (at most two) patients/residents for their twice weekly half-day experience spread across a two-week period. It was interesting to hear the nursing assistants critique of the student nurse experience. As they perceived it, playing the piano for a resident had nothing to do with real care. Some directors of nursing had the courage to terminate the clinical campus affiliation based on their conclusion that this was a wholly inadequate way to use the facility and learn about care of the elderly.

The clinical campus affiliation continued in many facilities, however, and was a fragile pipeline for the nursing home to potential recruitment of new graduates. In some affiliate arrangements, the nursing home was not a passive partner. Faculty offered to present one or two classes to the nursing staff. The library facilities of the nursing school were made available to the nursing home; videotapes were shared. In no case, however, did nursing home professional nursing staff do 'active' teaching with the students, e.g., demonstrating a technique; acting as classroom discussion leader. The only other role of the nursing home in clinical affiliation was as a rich source of data for research with a captive population. Prior to the Teaching Nursing Home Project (TNH) and the Community College Nursing Home Project (CCNHP), the nursing home was not construed as an "educational lab"—which it truly is or could be.

Whatever "education" that is taking place within long-term care institutions tends to be driven by regulations, i.e., OBRA '87, the minimum data set (MDS), the mandatory resident assessment-to-care plan data collection and analyses, and protocols for restraint reduction. Few, if any, initiatives to identify the learning needs *and* interests of the staff are undertaken. Many inservice instructors lack the fundamentals about principles of adult learning and evaluation of teaching.

External Education Initiatives

There are two types of external programs that provided "education" in institutional long-term care: oblique and direct. The *oblique* educational initiative comes about through scholarships and grants to nursing home staff who want to move along on the career ladder, e.g., Project LINC, the VA Program, the National Foundation for LTC grant, medical industry grants. With the exception of Project LINC, there is no stipulation that the student has to return to work in the long-term care setting. This requirement was often waived for Project LINC students as long as they worked in some kind of health care setting after graduation. In some cases, the "payback" was a cash return by the student, after graduation. In general, these projects provided manpower, not brain power. There were no identified monies for advanced clinical practice education. Critique of these programs was focused on the fact that their goal was retention of nurses, but not necessarily for long-term care. Improving the quality of care of the elderly was never an identified goal. The only other type of oblique educational initiative that comes to mind is the nursing home as research site.

The *direct* external initiative was in affiliation with hospital/university medical centers (NIA) and with schools of nursing (TNH, CCNHP). Broad objectives of these affiliate programs appeared to be *macro* and *micro*. From the larger view, the goals were: independence for as many older people as possible; quality of care/outcomes in long-term care (i.e., gerontological nursing science); increased knowledge about aging and geriatrics; and social policy decisions secondary to research. At the micro level, a direct educational affiliation—usually with a medical school—used the nursing home as a site for physician (and physician assistant) training and research in diagnosis, treatment, and case management. Graduate programs in advanced nursing, in either a managerial or clinical track, used the nursing home site to demonstrate and teach the pivotal role of nursing in care of the elderly. Very often, the nursing home provided a preceptor for the graduate student; faculty came to the site in varying frequencies. A critical weakness in these programs was the lack of preparation and guidance for the preceptor role.

The only other objective of affiliate educational programs was *cost containment*, relative to delivery of long-term institutional care. This goal had some interesting permutations. It was clearly demonstrated in some affiliate projects, like the TNH, which placed geriatric nurse practitioner (GNP) students in nursing homes, that health care system costs were reduced. For example, residents who would have been transferred to the hospital were managed in the nursing home. If the resident was transferred to acute care, the length of stay was shorter because the resident returned sooner to the nursing home because of the GNPs monitoring of care. Bladder and bowel retraining programs, as well as some behavioral interventions, were initiated by the GNPs with qualitative improvement in resident status. This 'improvement' was also measurable in dollars, i.e., it costs less to care for a continent resident than an incontinent resident *even if* maintaining continency required staff assistance for toileting more frequently. In New York State, a RUG-reimbursed state, (Research Utiligation Group) the return of the resident to the nursing home from the hospital more quickly had a perverse effect on overall revenues. Why? Because nursing homes are reimbursed for holding the (empty) bed; for guaranteeing that the Medicaid resident could return to the facility (within 20 days). A shorter bedhold meant a reduced profit margin for the facility even though system costs for hospitalization were reduced.

The role and benefits of advanced clinical practice specialists were well demonstrated by the TNH project. A secondary gain was that nursing home nurses had the opportunity to interact with colleagues who were moving along the career track *and* appeared to be practicing with greater assurance and autonomy. The GNPs were role models, in many cases. There are reports that some nurses chose to become "physician extenders" by selecting the physician assistant route. There is no data which indicates if these nurses returned to long-term care for practice, after graduation.

Problems encountered with educational affiliation/articulation programs were faculty preparedness and faculty misperception of the nursing home's needs—and support. These issues would have to be clarified before any joint venture or articulated program. Some nursing homes employ part-time nurses during peak summer vacation months. The full-time equivalent (FTE) dollars are set aside in the budget for this temporary staff to cover vacation allowance. If a school of nursing was interested in providing nursing home experience for (some of) the faculty, this kind of employment opportunity might well serve the faculty as well as the nursing facility.

Decisions about Policy and Funding for
Educational Alternatives

To make decisions about education articulation programs and their financial support, several issues need to be addressed.

1. What is the long-term care setting for which the educational program is being targeted? What is the "degree of fit" between the philosophy of the school of nursing and the mission and philosophy of the nursing home? Is there an *operational definition of a long-term care facility*, or long-term care, that directs the thrust of the educational venture—for both parties, i.e., nursing home and school? Four types of nursing home setting prevail:

   a. Mini-hospital

   b. Rehabilitation Center

   c. Hospice

   d. A place for frail elderly.

It is important that the dean and faculty 'know' the mind and mission set of the nursing home through which education for nursing students—and facility staff—will be exercised.

There are also diverse practice and care delivery models, theories (and non-theories) of nursing, and nursing organizational structures which prevail in all nursing homes. Again, is there congruency between the school of nursing and the nursing home? Does the articulation plan include a proposal to change the way nursing care is delivered in the nursing home? Will faculty and student practice differ radically from the nursing delivery style in the nursing home? These aspects should be addressed before an articulation decision is reached. What does *continuity of care* mean to the nursing home staff and to the nursing school? Does it only happen in the day care center? One has to be assured that the makers and shakers of the articulation project are speaking a common language.

2. Is the goal of the education articulation program the 'real' or the 'ideal' long-term care setting and practice model. For example, what kind of staff education is necessary for the nursing home with a staffing waiver in effect, i.e., that there does not have to be licensed staff on duty 24 hours. What is the role and positioning of the various nursing staff in the nursing home? What are the professed educational needs and *readiness to learn* of the staff? Was the importance of each learning objective rated, e.g., "definitely important, probably important, important, probably not important, definitely not important." Is the role and relationship of the certified nurse assistant and the "nurse team" really understood by the educators? Can education help a nursing director and/or administrator

understand if it is dysfunctional or ineffective with respect to quality of care outcomes? How does a school of nursing judge 'readiness to participate' by a long-term care facility in a joint education venture?

3. What will the 'educated' performance look like? What competencies can the nursing home expect of its staff as a result of the education articulation? Who participated in drawing up this list; did it come from a national organization; is there room for 'local' modification? What changes will there be in quality of care outcomes? What will the changes be in staff satisfaction with their own work, with the care they have given? Can we measure this in a meaningful way? Finally, what are the costs of achieving the competency?

4. Faculty availability, interest, preparedness; role model attributes. Joint practice models should be explored but it should be a two-way street, i.e., faculty spends time at the nursing facility and staff spends time at school (adjunct faculty position?). Caution must be taken to insure that joint practice care/case management between faculty and staff is collaborative care-giving and not 'parallel play.' Is it possible that a nursing home can choose the faculty person it wishes to be on premises, with students, or is there no choice? How is faculty development analyzed with respect to attitude, interest, and knowledge in gerontological nursing? More should be done with using nursing home nurses as adjunct faculty; teach them how to teach. After all, a good portion of their time is spent teaching residents and family, and teaching staff.

5. What learning experiences will best achieve the educational goals and performance objectives—for the students and the nursing home staff? What is the match between the curriculum and the experience within the nursing home which it has to offer? Should mastery of gerontological nursing, theory and practice, be evident (and tested) at a point in time or is the accrual of this knowledge and skills a cumulative effect, tested and seen only by very rudimentary measures?

6. The "interdisciplinary team" approach to resident assessment, care planning, intervention, and evaluation is part of OBRA '87 and incorporated into the resident's rights, as well as the nursing home's philosophy of care/services. How can the nursing home be assured that this principle is understood by faculty such that they can model and teach it to nursing students? The interdisciplinary team method is more than a weekly or monthly meeting to fill out reams of paper. It is a

method of communication, respect, and recognition that different professionals or therapeutic regimens may take precedence at different points in a resident's world of care needs—yet, all clinical services support that proximate goal while continuing to work and support each other for the distal goals.

Policy and program implications were well explicated by Aiken in her description of the teaching nursing home program contract affiliations. These included:

1. Joint mission statement of the philosophy and goals of the education articulation.
2. A steering committee composed of members from both venues.
3. Resources and responsibilities of each part.
4. A description of the decision-making process.
5. Credentials and qualifications of the teaching staff, both academic and institutional.
6. Mechanisms to evaluate effectiveness relative to program goals.
7. Reciprocal relationships; shared resources; exchanged resources.
8. Student nurse placement decisions.
9. Nursing assistant education; career track advisement.
10. Role and responsibility of the nursing home administrator and dean of the school of nursing.

Funding implications, or more prosaically put, the cost of the education articulation could be addressed in several ways. Faculty practice is one way to cover nursing home staff on leave or on an unpaid day off (to attend class); the nurse's salary covers the faculty salary for the day. There is an urgent need to demonstrate the cost and benefit of advanced nursing practice/practitioners in long-term care. Are nurses less interested in geriatric nursing as a reflection of reimbursement, salary, and minuscule tuition reimbursement policies? What is the owner/administrator predilection for innovation, risk-taking?

One funding approach that could be tried is to persuade the regulatory agency in the region to waive the formal resident assessment (mandated by OBRA '87) for one year. Data is showing, as it has for years, even prior to the OBRA resident assessment tool, that resident acuity (case mix index) remains essentially the same across time. Use the salary of the utilization review nurse to defray the costs of staff education. The CHAP experience is instructive; one can take on government and bureaucracy and win some points. Another funding proposal is a kind of incentive program: demonstrate that there are reduced system costs (e.g., hospitalization, pressure sore development) when advanced practice clinicians are in the nursing home sector. System savings could be 'returned' to the nursing home to cover the costs of staff education/advancement for improved clinical outcomes.

REFERENCES

Aiken, L. M. (1988). The Robert Wood Johnson Foundation Teaching Nursing Homes: Implications for improving care, education, and research. Ch. 3. In *Teaching Nursing Homes. The Nursing Perspective*, Small, N. R. & Walsh, M. B., Eds. Maryland: National Health Publishing.

Bowers, B., & Becker, M. (1992). Nurse's aides in nursing homes: The relationship between organization and quality. *The Gerontologist, 32*, (3).

Hanson, H. A., & Waters, V. (1991). Sequence of curriculum change in gerontology: Faculty first. *Nursing & Health Care, 12* (10).

Putney, K. A. et al. (1992). Case management in long-term care: New directions for professional nursing. *Journal of Gerontological Nursing, 16* (12).

Smyer, M. et al. (1992). Improving nursing home care through training and job redesign. *The Gerontologist, 32* (3).

Stephany, T. M. (1991). Who says new grads should practice in hospitals? *Nursing & Health Care, 12* (9).

Tagliareni, E. et al. (1991). Participatory clinical education. Reconceptualizing the clinical learning environment. *Nursing & Health Care, 12* (5).

Teaching Nursing Homes. The Nursing Perspective. (1988). Small, N. R. & Walsh, M. B., Eds. Maryland: National Health Publishing.

10

Response to: "Policy and Funding Implications of Programs Providing Education in Long-Term Care Institutions"

Gary Filerman

I considered the general question of long-term care educational policy and thought about it in the context of the previous papers and discussions. There have been many comments about the opportunity of the times. The context is the impending reform of "the system." I think the bottom line issue is: How will long-term care nursing education position itself in the context of reform? And with what deliberate speed, "much to do about nothing" and with what orderly process can we be sure that this discussion isn't because we missed the train? That is what really concerns me.

It is very tempting to take a wait and see position because there are so many varied proposals being circulated. It is more comfortable and less risky to stay back from the skirmish of getting involved in the fundamental reform debate because you don't want to be identified with one side or the other and, therefore, run the risk of somehow losing out. Here and now, we can identify enough of the parameters of the emerging consensus to be able to articulate a policy framework for long-term care nursing education which fits well with the direction in which the reform policy development process is moving.

I am talking about *structural reform* as opposed to most discussions about access and finance. Sooner rather than later, the reform discussion must focus on the structural issues of quality, capacity, and productivity of the health care system. It is at that level that the interests of long-term care nursing education are embedded in the reform process. That is the level of analysis to which we need to address ourselves. I think that policy can be built with a high degree of confidence around the following *premises of reform:*

First, as we have all agreed, reform is ultimately going to recognize the central role of integrated systems serving populations that are either defined by geography or by employment. That is managed care. Secondly, the systems that are at the core will go through predictable stages of growth. The first stage is now, in which we see a heterogeneous group of systems, some hospital systems, some managed care systems. In the second stage, we will see a convergence of systems around primary care, because of the payment system and other necessary elements of reform policy. At the third stage, there will be *a shift from primary care to primary health care* as a central focus.

The distinction is critically important because primary care is a passive concept. Primary health care is a proactive concept. It defines a totally different operating philosophy for the delivery of services in which the service system recognizes its economic stake in reducing risk and improving the health status of the population. There will be a fundamental shift to a managerial epidemiological perspective. Those are predictable stages of organization development in the process of reforming the structure.

Third, the core of the systems will be hospitals, group practices, or some combination of the two. The hospital role is being redefined in the ways which have been discussed earlier. The less clearly recognized option for system leadership is the group practice. My fourth premise is that control of the systems will be embedded in the groups or in free-standing control centers, sort of a corporate headquarters concept. Fifth, the evolution of group practice has become a generational phenomenon. Young physicians are moving toward groups. Groups are going to be responsible for quality of care and they are going to develop the same kind of internal quality control mechanisms that we now associate with hospitals. The reason that is germane to this discussion, is that with global budgeting or capitation, or much more broadly defined reimbursement systems, groups are going to have a lot of incentives to become truly multi-disciplinary. The groups, plus community health centers and all kinds of managed care permutations that are developed within this framework will become primary, clinical teaching sites. There is increasing pressure on medical education to move in that direction today, and to be ahead of the curve. The policy framework pursued here must recognize and move in that direction.

The sixth parameter of reform is the revaluation of primary care. There is a very consequential opportunity for nursing to lead in defining how primary care integrates with long-term care in the context of system reform. The existing definitions of primary care are fuzzy, and they don't meet the needs of the emerging structure. Primary care is a fuzzy concept, in part, because it is getting sexy for every specialty to claim that is what they do. That creates a kind of policy vacuum which is an opportunity for nursing to make a very critical contribution.

Seventh, the reform process is going to have to address health manpower policy. It is going to be influenced strongly by the product of the Pew Commission on the future of the health professions. The Commission's first report has received an immense amount of attention by the educational and policy establishment, and it is going to get a lot of attention in Congress. This is not just another report that is going to go on the shelf. Timing is everything. The fact is that congressional staff's see current health manpower policy as tired, as essentially propped up by political clout, and they are looking for an alternative approach. Just at the right time, here is this report (i.e., the Pew Report) which has powerful legitimacy. Therefore, it is going to get a lot of attention. Even if the Pew trusts do not put their financial clout behind making the reports influential, the policy process will do it for them. Nursing must attach itself to that vehicle and direct the policy interpretation in the most constructive fashion.

My eighth point is that comprehensive health systems are large and getting larger. Large enterprises learn how to optimize their human resource investment. They are very different from independent, small units. I don't care if it is a six-hundred-bed hospital, or a nursing home, or a VA; it is a very different human resource allocation enterprise than an integrated system. They will have sufficient critical mass to create *human resource markets.* If the educational establishment does not produce what they need, they will "grow their own." There is every reason to look forward to the Kaiser College of Health Sciences or to Mercy College becoming the captive of the Mercy system, and so on. They're thinking about it. They are going to do it. The nursing education establishment will have no control over that. It is something that has happened in industry to a great extent. The licensure system that recognizes the legitimacy of educational institutions is becoming much more flexible. That is why we have an Arthur D. Little College of Business, and Massachusetts General Hospital, licensed as degree granting institutions.

We must realize that industry, large scale enterprises, are spending more money on their internal education system than they are spending on collegiate level instruction. I am not talking about short courses. I am referring to industries which are spending more on college-level internal education than the budgets of all the colleges and universities in the country combined. It reflects a set of judgments which are being made about *how best to invest human resource development capital.*

Others will count these premises differently, but in my judgment those are the "hooks" of a public policy framework. The long-term care nursing reform agenda has to be fashioned to comprehensively address several things. First, it must address all of the targets for change, not only federal finance and manpower legislation. They include the role of systems, the role of groups in primary care, clinical education, State Board responsibilities, accreditation, and the long-term care industry, among others. All of those targets are within the scope of the policy which nursing addresses. Secondly, I think you should define the scope of long-term care as Sr. Rosemary Donley did, showing how primary nursing care relates directly to that definition. Do it in very clear terms, not leaving any assumptions to the readers. Show how the scope of long-term care, defined in those terms, drives the needs in terms of numbers of nurses, curriculum reform, cost of education, and reform of each of the targets of change that I have identified.

Third, and this is the tough one, curriculum and faculty reform has got to be addressed with powerful candor. You've got to get the attention of critical audiences, including the faculties, and create a sense of urgency even at the risk of creating a split within the ranks. This is where the rubber band hits the road. If you don't take advantage of the urgency of reform and the turbulence of the time, nursing is going to be left behind. The fact of life is you can't teach what you don't know. There is a lot of positioning and posturing that we all know exactly what to teach and we're just not appreciated. But we have acknowledged around this table that that is not the case, and it should be acknowledged publicly. That is going to earn nursing support because the public and policy makers are recognizing inadequacies. If you are candid and you face the inadequacies directly, you will get support to solve those problems.

Fourth, long-term care nursing should develop a crisp research agenda that addresses the barriers to implementing reform for adequate long-term care, and to improving learning about long-term care. It is no longer sufficient to simply angle for more money for nursing research: "just give us more and we're going to do good." Now is the time to seek support to solve problems that really address society's long-term care needs in the context of reform, and to be sharply focused.

Nursing education's reform policy should address the educational partnership with service delivery systems. It is time to redefine the meaning of partnership. Total partnership is the only way that education and service are going to grow together as the service structure evolves through the reform process. *Total Quality Management (TQM) mandates total collaboration between education which is a supplier and the systems which are the purchasers.* Adopt that mentality. The faculty have to get away from their computer screens and move out into the systems. Each school is going to have to create a special relationship with one or more systems. Encourage schools to find a partner system; get faculty involved in research into the system's problems—in service, is system education, so that it is a two-way learning process. The students and faculty in other systems will ultimately benefit. But schools cannot shy away from the necessity of creating special relationships with at least one system, getting to know it very well over time, and shaping its people to meet the school's needs and vice versa.

Finally, let us address the question: what is the real constituency for long-term care nursing education? Who are the stakeholders in this process? Who are the stakeholders in the adequacy of nursing competencies in this arena? It is probably a much broader group than we tend to think. Aggressively seek the support of those stakeholders in pursuing the fulfillment of this educational policy. But again, a very broadly defined educational policy. It isn't just the Feds; it's the States, it's the chains; it's all of those targets of opportunity integrated within one policy framework. This will get us closest to meeting the needs of long-term care education.

Appendix A

Competencies of the Baccalaureate and Higher Degree Nursing Graduate

In the last decade of the 20th century, nursing finds itself as an active participant in the changing health care delivery system. The role of the nurse has changed in response to demographics, to cost containment policies, to the decreased rate of mortality, and to the increase in numbers of citizens afflicted with chronic conditions. Graduates from baccalaureate programs are entering a practice arena where 60 to 80 percent of clients across the continuum of care are over age 65 years and increasingly over age 85. Older persons over the age of 85 years constitute the fastest growing segment of the older population, and this age group consumes a large portion of health care resources both in institutional care and in community-based care.

If the baccalaureate graduate is educated to assume a leadership role, what knowledge and skills are required to begin practice in the field of gerontologic nursing? There is agreement among nursing leaders in practice, education, and administration that there is a critical need to identify minimum gerontologic nursing skills and knowledge that can be expected of beginning baccalaureate nursing graduates.

This question has been addressed in several publications over the past several years but there has not been a consensus of gerontologic

Note: Competencies of the Baccalaureate and Higher Degree Nursing Graduate were previously published in *Gerontology in the Nursing Curriculum*, copyright © 1992, National League for Nursing Press.

nursing leaders from practice and from administration as to what are realistic, minimum expectations for beginning practice. In the same quandary are nurse educators who have not reached agreement on what are the minimum, realistic objectives for student learning given curriculum constraints. This issue was first addressed at Georgetown University School of Nursing as a part of the three-year project, Gerontologic Nursing Education Continuing Care (GRNECC) Project, funded by the Division of Nursing, United States Public Health Service (USPHS), Department of Health and Human Services (DHHS). The project faculty recognized the critical need to have gerontologic nursing competencies identified by national gerontologic nursing leaders.

With corporate funding and university support, the National Invitational Consensus Conference to Identify Gerontologic Nursing Competencies for Baccalaureate Graduates was convened on October 8 and 9, 1990, at Georgetown University. Eighteen leaders in gerontologic nursing practice, administration, and education were invited to donate two days to intensive, group-facilitated consensus building.

The consensus workshop was opened by a keynote address by Dr. Thelma Wells who emphasized the need for the identification of gerontologic nursing competencies for various levels of nursing education. Dr. Wells recounted the historical attempts to identify and the failure to gain acceptance of these competencies. The consultant for competency identification, Dr. Mary K. Stull, used a modified nominal group process to facilitate the attainment of the conference goal: consensus. The participants were divided into three groups with an equal mix of practitioners, administrators, and educators in each group. The organizing factor for the three working sessions was the nursing process, with participants identifying the essential knowledge for gerontologic nursing and developing desired attributes of nurses caring for older persons. The conference ended with participants expressing optimism that indeed a significant milestone for gerontologic nursing had occurred. They also agreed to continue to volunteer their time for the necessary validation of the work of the conference.

The first draft of the identified competencies was circulated to participants for confirmation of content and intent; the second draft was for leveling between baccalaureate and master's (gerontologic nursing specialization) preparation.

The competencies identified are not inclusive of all competencies for baccalaureate graduates which are identified in most curricula and in *Essentials of Baccalaureate Education* (AACN, 1986) as applicable "across the life span." Only those competencies which warrant specific emphasis on the older person are included in this document.

This final document is a refinement of comments from participants edited by GRNECC project personnel.

Norma R. Small, PhD, RN, Project Director
Mary Burke, DNSc, RN
Marjorie Maddox, EdD, RN
Mary K. Stull, PhD, RN, Consultant

Georgetown University
Washington, DC
May 1991

Competency Statements
Associate Degree Graduates

COMPETENCIES BEST TAUGHT IN THE NURSING HOME

Perform Assessment of Resident

Assesses current mental status.

Assesses functional (ADL & instrumental) abilities.

Differentiates normal aging process from disease process.

Recognizes age-related differences in disease processes.

Values goals that maintain optimal functional ability.

Practice Rehabilitation Nursing Skills

Defines restorative goals.

Elicits active participation of resident in restorative program.

Facilitates choices to decrease learned helplessness.

Promotes independence of ADLs.

Initiates bowel and bladder training.

Implements contracture-prevention methods.

Evaluates effectiveness of restorative programs.

Implements group therapies (e.g., reality orientation, memory enhancement, reminiscing).

Manage the Living Environment

Allows resident to continue previous lifestyle to degree possible.

Provides comfortable home-like environment for socialization.

Plans room arrangement to facilitate resident needs.

Reduces environmental stress (e.g., noises, isolation, lighting, roommate).

Provides opportunities for expression of ethnic and cultural practice for residents.

Provides for sexual expression of residents.

Initiates interventions to deal with combative residents.

Assists families to cope with unrealistic expectations, guilt, anger.

Exhibit Management Skills

Adopts leadership style appropriate to situation.

Delegates appropriately.

Resolves problems utilizing problem-solving skills over an extended period of time.

Updates plan of care.

Competency Statements
Baccalaureate Graduates

PROFESSIONAL PRACTICE

1.0 When providing nursing care to older persons, their significant others and community, the baccalaureate graduate will:

    1.1   Use a nursing practice theory to guide nursing care.

    1.2   Identify aging theories germane to nursing.

    1.3   Recognize normal changes of aging (psychological, physical, social, cultural, and spiritual).

    1.4   Identify health problems commonly found in older persons.

    1.5   Recognize atypical presentations of multiple pathological responses.

    1.6   Recognize the altered effects of drugs and multiple treatment modalities.

    1.7   Employ family systems theory.

    1.8   Incorporate bioethical principles.

    1.9   Apply the standards of gerontologic nursing practice.

    1.10 Recognize economic factors which influence nursing care of older persons.

    1.11 Discuss pertinent gerontologic nursing research findings.

    1.12 Apply pertinent geriatric/gerontology research findings.

1.13 Use knowledge of cultural and ethnic differences.

1.14 Demonstrate therapeutic communication skills which take into consideration normal aging and common pathological changes in aging.

2.0 When coordinating the human and material resources for the provision of care for older persons, their significant others and community, the baccalaureate graduate will:

2.1 Identify health care system resources and financing for the provision of care.

2.2 Discuss management theory.

2.3 Use concepts of delegation, negotiation, and collaboration.

2.4 Recognize the need for case management across the continuum of care.

2.5 Discuss the supervision needed for nursing and ancillary personnel.

2.6 Describe management skills involved in the coordination of care.

3.0 When demonstrating accountability for own gerontological nursing practice, the baccalaureate graduate will:

3.1 Use standards of gerontologic nursing practice.

3.2 Use legal and regulatory parameters of practice.

3.3 Advocate for the older client's rights regarding dignity, access to care, and conservation of physical, emotional and material resources.

3.4 Demonstrate responsibility for professional practice and the development of gerontologic nursing by participating in peer review.

3.5 Develop a sensitivity to older persons as unique individuals.

3.6 Demonstrate creativity in adapting nursing care to the needs of older persons.

3.7 Demonstrate flexibility in response to conflicting values when providing nursing care to older persons and their families.

3.8 Develop a sense of confidence in professional practice with older persons and their families.

3.9 Demonstrate acceptance of the older person regardless of health state.

3.10 Demonstrate a sense of humor and the ability to laugh at oneself and with others.

3.11 Demonstrate empathy for the older person during transitions, e.g., health, housing, socio-economic status.

NURSING PROCESS

Assessment:

4.0 When assessing older persons, their significant others and community, the baccalaureate graduate will:

4.1 Differentiate normal aging from pathological change.

4.2 Recognize the importance of appropriate theory, knowledge, and research needed to guide the assessment of older persons.

4.3 Demonstrate interviewing skills which take into account normal and common pathological changes of aging.

4.4 Use standardized assessment procedures and tools to assess physical, psychological, cognitive, social, spiritual strengths and deficits.

4.5 Adapt the use of various health assessment tools/procedures/ equipment to meet the needs of older persons.

4.6 Identify the structure and dynamics of caregiving.

4.7 Demonstrate the skills needed to assess physical, psychological, socio-economics, and functional status of older persons.

4.8 Demonstrate the assessment skills needed to identify areas of health promotion and disease prevention for older persons.

4.9 Determine appropriate nursing diagnoses.

4.10 Validate assessment data with client, family, significant others, and other members of the interdisciplinary team.

Planning:

5.0 When planning nursing care for older persons, their significant others and community, the baccalaureate graduate will:

    5.1 Develop mutual goals with client and/or family that are realistic and measurable.

    5.2 Incorporate legal and regulatory requirements.

    5.3 Identify various social support systems available.

    5.4 Develop health promotion strategies appropriate to formulated goals.

    5.5 Identify mutually agreed upon, realistic priorities.

    5.6 Recognize the importance of using theory, research findings, and the standards of gerontologic nursing practice.

    5.7 Demonstrate an appreciation of client's values.

    5.8 Develop a plan of care within the client's socio-economic resources.

    5.9 Review the established plan of care with the client periodically to promote maximum involvement across the continuum of care.

    5.10 Recognize learning and teaching needs of care givers and older persons.

    5.11 Use consultation with interdisciplinary team members.

    5.12 Promote the attainment and maintenance of the highest level of health, well-being, quality of life and a peaceful death as defined by the older person and/or family/significant others.

Implementation:

6.0 When implementing a plan of care for older persons, their significant others and community, the baccalaureate graduate will:

    6.1 Use goal-oriented preventive, maintenance, restorative and comfort treatment modalities.

    6.2 Use appropriate teaching-learning techniques.

6.3 Suggest changes in the established plan of care in a timely manner.

6.4 Document nursing interventions in measurable terms that are useful and retrievable to nursing, interdisciplinary team members, and administrators.

6.5 Use the plan of care across the continuum of care.

6.6 Apply legal and ethical principles.

6.7 Apply gerontologic nursing research findings to interventions.

6.8 Promote independence.

6.9 Demonstrate respect for the autonomy, dignity and rights of older persons in health care decision-making.

Evaluation:

7.0 When evaluating the plan of care for older persons, their significant others and community, the baccalaureate graduate will:

7.1 Discuss outcomes in relation to interventions.

7.2 Compare and contrast outcomes with mutually agreed upon goals.

7.3 Identify ethical conflicts.

7.4 Document outcomes in relation to mutually agreed upon goals.

7.5 Appreciate the complexity in evaluating the total clinical picture of the older person.

7.6 Contribute to the interdisciplinary team evaluation.

7.7 Use professional standards of care and quality management criteria.

7.8 Discuss outcomes in relation to regulatory and reimbursement criteria.

Competency Statements
Master's Graduates

PROFESSIONAL PRACTICE

1.0 When providing nursing care to older persons, their significant others and community, the master's graduate will:

1.1 Compare and contrast nursing practice theories used to guide nursing care.

1.2 Analyze aging theories germane to the nursing care of older persons.

1.3 Evaluate normal changes of aging (psychological, physical, social, cultural, and spiritual).

1.4 Manage common health problems related to normal aging changes.

1.5 Evaluate atypical presentations of multiple pathological responses.

1.6 Examine the effects of drugs and multiple treatment modalities.

1.7 Apply family systems theory.

1.8 Apply bioethical principles.

1.9 Examine legal regulations related to nursing and health care.

1.10 Analyze economic factors which influence the nursing care of older persons.

1.11 Conduct gerontologic nursing research.

1.12 Evaluate geriatric/gerontology research findings.

1.13 Integrate the knowledge of cultural and ethnic differences.

1.14 Test therapeutic communication skills which take into consideration normal aging and common pathological changes in aging.

2.0 When coordinating human and material resources for the provision of care for older persons, their significant others and community, the master's graduate will:

2.1 Manage health care system resources and financing.

2.2 Use management theories to coordinate human and material resources.

2.3 Apply delegation, negotiation and collaboration strategies.

2.4 Use case management strategies across the continuum of care.

2.5 Provide the supervision needed for nursing and ancillary personnel.

2.6 Analyze management skills.

3.0 When demonstrating accountability for own gerontologic nursing practice, the master's graduate will:

3.1 Use standards of gerontologic nursing practice.

3.2 Propose additional legal and regulatory parameters for gerontologic nursing practice.

3.3 Organize individuals and groups to advocate for the older client's rights to dignity, access to care, and the conservation of physical, emotional and material resources.

3.4 Evaluate responsibility for professional practice and for the development of gerontologic nursing by participating in peer review.

3.5 Demonstrate a sensitivity to older persons as unique individuals.

3.6 Test creative adaptations of nursing care to the needs of older persons.

3.7 Analyze own flexibility in response to conflicting values when providing nursing care to older persons and their families.

3.8 Manage professional practice with older persons and their families with a sense of confidence.

3.9 Appraise own acceptance of the older person regardless of health state.

3.10 Examine the use of humor and the ability to laugh at oneself and with others.

3.11 Empathize with the older person during transitions, e.g., health, housing, socio-economic.

NURSING PROCESS

Assessment:

4.0 When assessing older persons, their significant others and community, the master's graduate will:

4.1 Test health assessment tools/instruments.

4.2 Discriminate normal aging from pathological states.

4.3 Analyze appropriate theory, knowledge and research needed to guide the assessment of older persons.

4.4 Analyze interviewing skills which take into account normal and common pathological changes of aging.

4.5 Design various health assessment tools/procedures/equipment to meet the needs of older persons.

4.6 Evaluate standardized assessment procedures and tools when assessing physical, psychological, cognitive, social, spiritual strengths and deficits.

4.7 Analyze the structure and dynamics of caregiving.

4.8 Examine the complexity of the interactions among the physical, psychological, socio-economic and functional processes of older persons.

4.9 Develop advanced assessment skills needed to identify the areas of health promotion and disease prevention for older persons.

4.10 Evaluate the appropriateness of nursing diagnoses based on the assessment of the health status of older persons.

4.11 Validate assessment data with client, family, significant others, and other members of the interdisciplinary team.

Planning:

5.0 When planning nursing care for older persons, their significant others and community, the master's graduate will:

   5.1 Synthesize assessment data and nursing diagnoses to establish goals and priorities.

   5.2 Formulate mutual goals with client and/or family that are realistic and measurable.

   5.3 Establish mutually agreed upon goals with realistic priorities.

   5.4 Plan health promotion strategies appropriate to formulated goals and the plan of care.

   5.5 Analyze legal and regulatory implications.

   5.6 Validate available social support systems.

   5.7 Analyze ethical principles.

   5.8 Develop standards for gerontologic nursing practice.

   5.9 Integrate theory, research findings, and the standards of gerontologic nursing practice when establishing a plan of care for older persons.

   5.10 Validate client's values.

   5.11 Evaluate client's socioeconomic resources.

   5.12 Redesign plan of care with the client periodically to promote maximum involvement across the continuum of care.

   5.13 Validate the learning mode and teaching needs of care givers and the older persons.

   5.14 Consult with interdisciplinary team members when establishing a plan of care.

   5.15 Design plan of care which promotes the attainment and maintenance of health, well-being, quality of life and a peaceful death as defined by the older person and/or family/significant others.

Implementation:

6.0 When implementing a plan of care with older persons, their significant others and community, the master's graduate will:

    6.1 Evaluate treatment modalities in relation to preventive, maintenance, restorative and comfort needs of the older person.

    6.2 Incorporate the knowledge of age related changes, altered responses to diseases, nursing interventions, pharmacological interventions, medical interventions.

    6.3 Incorporate appropriate teaching-learning theory and techniques into a plan of care.

    6.4 Alter the plan of care based on changing needs of the older client.

    6.5 Negotiate changes in the established plan of care in a timely manner.

    6.6 Document nursing interventions in measurable terms that are useful and retrievable to nursing, interdisciplinary team members, and administrators.

    6.7 Validate the plan of care with older persons across the continuum of care.

    6.8 Integrate legal and ethical principles in clinical decision-making.

    6.9 Evaluate gerontologic nursing research findings.

    6.10 Advocate for promotion of independence in the plan of care.

    6.11 Promote the autonomy of older persons in health care decision-making.

Evaluation:

7.0 When evaluating the plan of care for older persons, their significant others and community, the master's graduate will:

    7.1 Evaluate outcomes in relation to mutually agreed upon goals.

    7.2 Synthesize all data in the evaluation of the total clinical picture of the older person.

7.3 Discuss ethical issues.

7.4 Design quality management criteria.

7.5 Evaluate standards of gerontologic nursing.

7.6 Critique regulatory and reimbursement requirements.

7.7 Use advanced knowledge of altered responses to diseases and to medical, pharmacological, and nursing interventions.

7.8 Contribute specialized knowledge to the interdisciplinary team regarding the evaluation of the plan of care.

7.9 Compare and contrast clinical outcomes with relevant research findings.

7.10 Evaluate outcomes based on professional standards of care and quality management criteria.

7.11 Evaluate outcomes in relation to regulatory and reimbursement criteria.

7.12 Evaluate the use of ethical principles in all components of the nursing process.

Appendix B

Minimum Competencies of Nursing Staff in LTC Facilities

Intended Usage: The following list represents minimum competencies that should be reviewed by both individuals seeking advancement in nursing education and by academic institutions as a basis for granting course waivers. Those individuals who demonstrate competency in any of the following ways should be able to petition academic institutions for credit waivers.

MINIMUM COMPETENCIES: CERTIFIED NURSE ASSISTANT

Purpose:

To perform non-professional direct resident care under the supervision of licensed, professional nursing staff; to provide the necessary care and service for residents that allows each to attain and maintain the highest practicable physical, mental, and psychosocial well being; to provide the necessary personal care and support of nursing service.

Requirements:

Certified Nursing Assistant and completion of 75-hour minimum nurse assistant training and certification in accordance with state and federal regulation.

Twelve-hour minimum continuing education requirement in accordance with state and federal regulation.

Ability to communicate.

Resident Rights

Knock when entering a resident's room.

Identify resident by wrist band.

Call residents by their proper name unless otherwise instructed.

Introduce yourself to residents.

Introduce staff and other residents to residents.

Treat residents with respect, dignity, and self-determination.

Inform residents of their rights.

Treat residents as individuals, offering choice and autonomy.

Provide privacy and confidentiality.

Encourage residents' participation in activities, resident groups, and community activities, and care planning.

Accommodate resident's preferences.

Offer assistance and respond to all requests.

Answer resident calls.

Keep nursing call system within reach of residents.

Report resident complaints.

Report any violations in mistreatment, neglect, or abuse.

Admission, Transfer, and Discharge

Prepare the resident's room for admission (i.e., make bed, prepare name tags, make available an admission kit, prepare and arrange necessary care items).

Greet and accompany resident.

Introduce residents to each other and resident to staff.

Make resident comfortable.

Mark and inventory resident's personal items.

Store and put away resident's personal items.

Transport and accompany residents during transfer or discharge.

Collect resident's personal belongings upon discharge.

Personal Care

Assist residents with bathing, dressing, grooming, dental/mouth care, nail and foot care, hair care.

Shave male residents as necessary and maintain cleanliness of female residents by making sure they are clean shaven.

Assist with perineal care.

Assist skin care and backrubs.

Assist residents with bladder and bowel care.

Assist residents with sensory stimulation (taste, hearing, smell, sight, touch) and ear and eye care.

Assist residents with positioning, transferring, and ambulation.

Transport residents.

Assist residents with evening care.

Make unoccupied and occupied beds.

Maintain the resident's environment.

Check residents frequently and as required. Report missing residents immediately to supervisor.

Keep nursing call system within reach of residents.

Nursing Care/Special Care

Assist with and assess changes in condition.

Participate in resident assessment and care planning as directed.

Check care plan to identify changes that have occurred.

Report all changes in resident condition to supervisor.

Where permitted by state regulation, provide functions as directed by the charge nurse or nurse supervisor: care of residents with catheters, nonsterile dressing and bandaging, vital signs, incontinence care, range of motion/restorative/rehabilitative care, enemas, specimen collection, care of residents with feeding tubes, ostomy care, diabetic testing and other urine testing.

Take and record intake and output.

Take and record resident height and weight.

Prepare residents for medical and nursing procedures.

Report and return all medications found in the resident's room to supervisor.

Assist with care of the comatose resident.

Assist with care of dying resident.

Provide post-mortem care as required.

Food and Dietary Services

Transport residents to/from meals.

Validate accuracy of resident's trays with dietary orders.

Serve trays to appropriate residents.

Prepare the resident for meals.

Identify all food items for residents. Assist with stimulating sense of smell and taste.

Assist with eating, drinking.

Assist resident with use of any assistive device.

After meals, ensure the area is clean and free of trays and food.

Prepare and offer water in water pitchers.

Offer and prepare snacks for residents.

Administer nourishments as ordered.

Infection Control and Safety

Wash hands as necessary and according to policies and procedures.

Isolation or infection precautions procedures (gown, glove, mask, double bagging).

Keep environment clean and safe (keep area dry, clean, odor-free, put supplies and equipment in their proper place).

At the end of your work period, check your work area and leave it clean and safe for residents and staff.

Use only equipment you have been trained to use.

Wipe off, clean, or disinfect equipment after use and as necessary.

Report defective equipment to supervisor.

Identify and report hazards to supervisor.

Report all accidents and emergencies to supervisor.

Maintain facility smoking policies. Identify and report violations.

Know the location of fire extinguishers.

Report to supervisor for instructions during an emergency.

Keep nursing call system in reach of residents.

Administrative and Personnel

Participate in orientation.

Use standard medical abbreviations for documentation.

Report to the nursing department.

Record and document all entries in resident flow charts/sheets, chart properly and in accordance with facility policies and resident care plan.

Receive assignment and report from the charge nurse or supervisor.

Use resident charge system for ancillary items and personal care equipment.

Follow work assignments.

Perform all assigned tasks.

Notify the facility when you will be late or absent.

Work with other staff and departments to care for residents and maintain facility policy.

Attend staff meetings.

Participate in inservice training activities.

Identify residents by wrist band.

Adhere to all personnel policies.

Participate and assist in survey inspections by authorized government officials.

Intended Usage: The following list represents minimum competencies that should be reviewed by both individuals seeking advancement in nursing education and by academic institutions as a basis for granting course waivers. Those individuals who demonstrate competency in any of the following ways should be able to petition academic institutions for credit waivers.

MINIMUM COMPETENCIES:
LICENSED PRACTICAL NURSE

Purpose:

To perform the highest quality of licensed and professional direct nursing care and service; to provide the necessary care and service for residents that allows each to attain and maintain the highest practicable physical, mental, and psychosocial well-being; to provide nursing service in accordance with state, federal, and facility policies and standards under the direction of a registered nurse, director of nursing service, or charge nurse; to supervise the activities of nursing assistants.

Requirements:

Licensed Practical Nurse in accordance with state and federal regulation.

Ability to communicate.

Resident Rights

Knock when entering a resident's room.

Identify resident by wrist band.

Call residents by their proper name unless otherwise instructed.

Introduce yourself to residents.

Introduce staff and other residents to residents.

Treat residents with respect, dignity, and self-determination.

Inform residents of their rights.

Treat residents as individuals, offering choice and autonomy.

Provide privacy and confidentiality.

Make the resident records available to that resident.

Make facility, federal, and/or state survey results available to residents for inspection.

Encourage resident's participation in activities, resident groups, and community activities, and care planning.

Work with therapy, activities, and other staff to ensure resident's participation and scheduling.

Accommodate resident's preferences.

Offer assistance and respond to all requests.

Keep nursing call system within reach of residents.

Answer resident calls.

Report resident complaints.

Report any violations in mistreatment, neglect, or abuse.

Notify the physician and legal representative or family member when there is an accident, a significant change in condition, or a need to alter treatment significantly.

Meet with or communicate with family members of residents and residents to discuss care and services.

Admission, Transfer, and Discharge

Receive and document admission orders by physician.

Coordinate preparation of the resident's room for admission.

Inform nursing staff of admissions, transfers, and discharges.

Greet residents and assist with facility orientation.

Introduce residents to each other and residents to staff.

Make resident comfortable.

Complete necessary documentation upon admission, discharge, or transfer.

Provide or assist with resident orientation at time of transfer or discharge.

Prepare the discharge summary and review and update discharge plan.

Assist with arranging transportation for discharged residents.

Resident Assessment and Care Planning

Participate in resident assessment: initial, quarterly, and annual reviews.

Assist with finalizing initial interdisciplinary assessment by 14th day of residency.

Identify and document changes in resident condition; participate in reassessment.

Participate in developing resident's care plan within seven days after comprehensive assessment is completed.

Review care plan daily.

Ensure that resident's care plan contains measurable goals, objectives, and timetables.

Update care plan as necessary and with any change in condition.

Make care plan available to nurse assistants and other departmental staff.

Encourage resident and resident's family to participate in care planning.

Nursing Care

Provide all necessary nursing care.

Identify nursing care needs in accordance with care plan goals.

Implement interventions in accordance with care plan.

Make decisions and recommendations with respect to nursing care.

Monitor nursing care; review; and modify.

Work with physician staff to ensure highest care: make rounds with physicians, follow doctors' orders, make recommendations to physician staff with respect to nursing and medical care, notify resident's physician in the case of an emergency or change in condition, coordinate all ordered laboratory, diagnostic, or clinical tests.

Where permitted by state regulation, administer and/or supervise nursing intervention: catheter, ostomy, nutrition and hydration, parenteral and enteral fluids, personal care, dressing/wound care, drainage, suctioning, packs/compresses, vital signs, incontinence care, bowel or bladder training, range of motion/restorative/rehabilitative care, prosthesis care, enemas, specimen collection, nasogastric/tube feeding, diabetic testing and other laboratory/medical testing, intake and output, height and weight, intravenous therapy, and others as required.

Prepare residents for medical procedures.

Provide care of the comatose resident.

Provide care of dying resident.

Provide post-mortem care as required.

Special Care

Participate in facility's quality assurance, quality improvement program as directed.

Drug and Medication Administration

Prepare, administer and document medication administration.

Identify resident and ensure medication prescribed is administered to the right resident.

Identify, document, report any adverse side effects.

Administer medication as prescribed by the physician.

Use nursing judgment to administer over-the-counter medications and treatments; document as required.

Maintain and properly store drugs.

Maintain the security of narcotics and controlled drugs.

Properly document and administer narcotics and controlled drugs.

Dispose of drugs, medications, and administration devices (i.e., syringes) properly and in accordance with facility procedures and infection control policies.

Take blood.

Notify physician when orders are needed or need to be refilled.

Review medication administration records for accuracy and completeness.

Report any medication errors to nurse supervisor immediately.

Contact pharmacy for any missing medication when dispensed.

Monitor the administration of medications by residents who are self-administering drugs as defined by the care plan.

Participate in drug utilization review.

Infection Control and Safety

Assist in developing safety and sanitation policies and procedures.

Ensure that personnel under supervision comply with sanitation and safety policies and procedures.

Wash hands as necessary and according to policies and procedures.

Ensure that handwashing techniques are properly used by staff.

Administer isolation or infection precautions procedures (gown, glove, mask, double bagging, identification of contaminated waste, isolation signs).

Participate in facility's infection control program.

Keep environment clean and safe (keep area dry, clean, odor-free, put supplies and equipment in their proper place).

At the end of your work period, check your work area and leave it clean and safe for residents and staff.

Use only equipment you have been trained to use.

Demonstrate use of equipment to nurse assistant staff.

Ensure that staff under supervision use equipment as instructed and in a safe manner.

Report defective equipment to supervisor or maintenance department.

Make recommendations to supervisor of equipment and supplies needed.

Wipe off, clean, or disinfect equipment after use and as necessary.

Identify and report hazards.

Report all accidents and emergencies; document according to facility policies.

Maintain facility smoking policies. Identify and report violations.

Know the location of fire extinguishers.

Implement emergency procedures.

Keep nursing call system in reach of residents.

Charting and Documentation

Use standard medical abbreviations for documentation.

Document resident and nursing care in resident charts, flow charts/sheets, and care plans.

Maintain resident assessment and care plan in the resident's chart.

Sign portion of resident assessment for which you are responsible.

Record in the resident's chart nurse's progress notes for each resident on each shift.

Document any changes in condition and notify charge nurse.

Receive and document telephone orders from physicians.

Transcribe physician orders onto resident charts, cardex, medication cards, treatment plan, and care plan as needed.

Report results of all laboratory, diagnostic, or clinical tests to resident's physician.

Record change in resident's diet orders; distribute to dietary department.

Sign and date all records.

Administrative and Supervisory

Report to the nursing department.

Receive assignment and report from the nurse being relieved, charge nurse, or supervisor.

Conduct nursing rounds to ensure staff is complying with work assignments and performance standards.

Work with other nursing staff and other departments to ensure the highest care possible.

Give report to charge nurse, supervisor, or nurse relief staff.

Use resident charge system for ancillary items and personal care equipment.

Monitor use of nursing and ancillary items and recommend list of supplies needed; maintain adequate levels.

Review and make recommendations for the revision of facility's nursing policies and procedures.

Make recommendations to nursing supervisor, director of nursing, and administrator to improve care and services.

Ensure that personnel, residents, and visitors follow established facility policies.

Report any violations of resident mistreatment, neglect, or abuse.

Participate and assist in survey inspections by authorized government officials.

Work with nursing supervisor responsible for scheduling in planning shifts.

Inform supervisor when staff does not report.

Work to substitute for absent nursing staff.

Direct and supervise the work of nurse assistants.

Make assignments for nursing assistants.

Participate in performance evaluations for those whom they supervise.

Staff Development and Personnel

Participate in orientation.

Receive assignment and report from the charge nurse or supervisor.

Follow work assignments.

Perform all assigned tasks.

Notify the facility when you will be late or absent.

Work with other staff and departments to care for residents and maintain facility policy.

Attend staff meetings.

Participate in inservice training activities.

Maintain licensure.

Adhere to all personnel policies.

Intended Usage: The following list represents minimum competencies that should be reviewed by both individuals seeking advancement in nursing education and by academic institutions as a basis for granting course waivers. Those individuals who demonstrate competency in any of the following ways should be able to petition academic institutions for credit waivers.

MINIMUM COMPETENCIES: REGISTERED NURSE

Purpose:

To perform the highest quality of licensed and professional direct nursing care and service; to provide the necessary care and service for residents that allows each to attain and maintain the highest practicable physical, mental, and psychosocial well-being; to provide nursing service in accordance with state, federal, and facility policies and standards; to supervise the activities of nursing assistants.

Requirements:

Licensed Registered Nurse in accordance with state and federal regulation.
Ability to communicate.

Resident Rights

Knock when entering a resident's room.
Identify resident by wrist band.
Call residents by their proper name unless otherwise instructed.
Introduce yourself to residents.
Introduce staff and other residents to residents.
Treat residents with respect, dignity, and self-determination.
Inform residents of their rights.
Treat residents as individuals, offering choice and autonomy.
Provide privacy and confidentiality.
Make the resident records available to that resident.
Make facility, federal, and/or state survey results available to residents for inspection.

Encourage resident's participation in activities, resident groups, and community activities, and care planning.

Work with therapy, activities, and other staff to ensure resident's participation and scheduling.

Accommodate resident's preferences.

Offer assistance and respond to all requests.

Answer resident calls.

Keep nursing call system within reach of residents.

Report resident complaints.

Report any violations in mistreatment, neglect, or abuse.

Notify the physician and legal representative or family member when there is an accident, a significant change in condition, or a need to alter treatment significantly.

Meet with or communicate with family members of residents and residents to discuss care and services.

Admission, Transfer, and Discharge

Receive and document admission orders by physician.

Coordinate preparation of the resident's room for admission.

Greet residents and assist with facility orientation.

Inform nursing staff of admissions, transfers, and discharges.

Introduce residents to each other and residents to staff.

Make resident comfortable.

Complete necessary documentation upon admission, discharge, or transfer.

Provide or assist with resident orientation at time of transfer or discharge.

Prepare the discharge summary and review and update discharge plan.

Assist with arranging transportation for discharged residents.

Resident Assessment and Care Planning

Coordinate and/or participate in resident assessment: initial, quarterly, and annual reviews.

Complete initial assessment after significant change in condition.

Identify and document changes in resident condition.

Complete interdisciplinary assessment by 14th day of residency.

Prepare and complete care plan seven days after comprehensive assessment is conducted.

Review care plan daily.

Ensure that resident's care plan contains measurable goals, objectives, and timetables.

Update care plan as necessary and with any change in condition.

Make care plan available to nurse assistants and other departmental staff.

Encourage resident and resident's family to participate in care planning.

Nursing Care

Provide all necessary nursing care.

Identify nursing care needs in accordance with care plan goals.

Implement interventions in accordance with care plan.

Make decisions and recommendations with respect to nursing care.

Monitor nursing care; review; and modify as needed.

Work with physician staff to ensure highest care: make rounds with physicians, follow doctor's orders, make recommendations to physician staff with respect to nursing and medical care, notify resident's physician in the case of an emergency or change in condition; request, arrange and coordinate all ordered laboratory, diagnostic, or clinical tests.

Administer and/or supervise nursing intervention: catheter, ostomy, nutrition and hydration, parenteral and enteral fluids, personal care, dressing/wound care, drainage, suctioning, packs/compresses, vital signs, incontinence care, bowel or bladder training, range of motion/restorative/rehabilitative care, prosthesis care, enemas, specimen collection, nasogastric/tube feeding, diabetic testing and other laboratory/medical testing, intake and output, height and weight, intravenous therapy, blood administration, and others as required.

Prepare residents for medical procedures.

Provide care of the comatose resident.

Provide care of dying resident.

Provide post-mortem care as required.

Special Care

Participate in facility's quality assurance, quality improvement program as directed.

Drug and Medication Administration

Prepare, administer and document medication administration.

Identify resident and ensure medication prescribed is administered to the right resident.

Identify, document, report any adverse side effects.

Administer medication as prescribed by the physician.

Use nursing judgment to administer over the counter medications and treatments; document as required.

Maintain and properly store drugs.

Maintain the security of narcotics and controlled drugs.

Properly document and administer narcotics and controlled drugs.

Dispose of drugs, medications, and administration devices (i.e., syringes) properly and in accordance with facility infection control policies and procedures.

Take blood.

Notify physician when orders are needed or need to be refilled.

Review medication administration records for accuracy and completeness.

Report any medication errors to nurse supervisor immediately.

Contact pharmacy for any missing medication when dispensed.

Monitor the administration of medications by residents who are self-administering drugs as defined by the care plan.

Conduct drug utilization review.

Infection Control and Safety

Assist in developing safety and sanitation policies and procedures.

Ensure that personnel under supervision comply with sanitation and safety policies and procedures.

Wash hands as necessary and according to policies and procedures.

Ensure that handwashing techniques are properly used by staff.

Administer isolation or infection precautions procedures (gown, glove, mask, double bagging, identification of contaminated waste, isolation signs).

Participate in facility's infection control program.

Keep environment clean and safe (keep area dry, clean, odor-free, put supplies and equipment in their proper place).

At the end of your work period, check your work area and leave it clean and safe for residents and staff.

Conduct or participate in safety drills and inspections.

Use only equipment you have been trained to use.

Demonstrate use of equipment to nurse assistant staff.

Ensure that staff under supervision use equipment as instructed and in a safe manner.

Report defective equipment to supervisor or maintenance department.

Make recommendations to supervisor of equipment and supplies needed on unit.

Wipe off, clean, or disinfect equipment after use and as necessary.

Identify and report hazards.

Report all accidents and emergencies; document according to facility policies; implement emergency procedures.

Maintain facility smoking policies. Identify and report violations.

Know the location of fire extinguishers.

Keep nursing call system in reach of residents.

Charting and Documentation

Use standard medical abbreviations for documentation.

Document resident and nursing care in resident charts, flow charts/sheets, and care plans.

Maintain resident assessment and care plan in the resident's chart.

Sign and certify the completion, or of that portion of the assessment in the resident's chart for which you are responsible.

Record in the resident's chart nurse's progress notes for each resident on each shift.

Document any changes in condition and notify charge nurse.

Receive and document telephone orders from physicians.

Transcribe physician orders onto resident charts, cardex, medication cards, treatment plan, and care plan as needed.

Report results of all laboratory, diagnostic, or clinical tests to resident's physician.

Record change in resident's diet orders; distribute to dietary department.

Sign and date all records.

Administrative and Supervisory

Report to the nursing department.

Receive assignment and report from the nurse being relieved, charge nurse, or supervisor.

Conduct nursing rounds to ensure staff is complying with work assignments and performance standards.

Work with other nursing staff and other departments to ensure the highest care possible and to ensure maintenance of facility procedures.

Give report to charge nurse, supervisor, or nurse relief staff.

Make assignments for nursing assistants.

Use resident charge system for ancillary items and personal care equipment.

Monitor use of nursing and ancillary items and recommend list of supplies needed; maintain adequate levels.

Review and make recommendations for the revision of facility's nursing policies and procedures.

Make recommendations to nursing supervisor, director of nursing, and administrator to improve care and services.

Ensure that personnel, residents, and visitors follow established facility policies.

Report any violations of resident mistreatment, neglect, or abuse.

Participate and assist in survey inspections by authorized government officials.

Work with nursing supervisor responsible for scheduling in planning shifts.

Inform supervisor when nursing staff does not report to work.

Work to substitute for absent nursing services staff.

Direct and supervise the work of nurse assistants.

Participate in performance evaluations for those whom they supervise.

Staff Development and Personnel

Participate in orientation.

Receive assignment and report from the charge nurse or supervisor.

Follow work assignments.

Perform all assigned tasks.

Notify the facility when you will be late or absent.

Work with other staff and departments to care for residents and maintain facility policy.

Attend staff meetings.

Participate in inservice training activities.

Maintain licensure.

Adhere to all personnel policies.

Appendix C

A Vision for Nursing Education Reform

*"Only to the degree that we become educated do we gain
relationships of depth and meaning to the encompassing world."*

J. Glenn Gray (1984)

A *Vision For Nursing Education* is a collective reflection of the ideas and
values of the members and Board of Governors of the National League for
Nursing who continue in the tradition of the past hundred years—
assuring, as Isabel Hampton Robb first wrote in 1893, that the graduates
of nursing programs are prepared to work with their heads, hearts and
hands in harmony.

This work was developed by listening to the conversations of NLN
members in council meetings, on programs and committees; reading their
literature and their resolutions; hearing their questions and their answers;
receiving the comments and suggestions of individual faculty, administrators of nursing services, and students.

This *Vision* is but one of the many with which the National League
for Nursing begins its second century of leadership in the interest of
"Health and The Public Trust."

Patricia Moccia, PhD, RN, FAAN
Chief Executive Officer
National League for Nursing
Boston, June 1993

A Vision for Nursing
Education Reform

Executive Summary

Nursing's vision for a health care system that ensures access, quality, and cost containment through a new approach to the delivery of care is within reach. The nursing education system required by that new approach must move quickly to provide adequate numbers of appropriately prepared nurses.

Successful implementation of nursing's approach to health care delivery requires:

1. Significant increases in the numbers of advanced nurse practitioners prepared to provide primary health care to communities and primary care services in group and interdisciplinary practices.

2. A shift in emphasis for all nursing education programs to ensure that all nurses—whatever their basic and graduate education and wherever they choose to practice—are prepared to function in a community-based, community focused health care system.

3. An increase in the numbers of community nursing centers and their increased utilization as model clinical sites for nursing students.

4. An increase in the number of nursing faculty prepared to teach for a community-based, community focused health care system.

5. A shift in emphasis for nursing research and an increase in the numbers of studies concerned with health promotion and disease prevention at the aggregate and community levels.

6. Targeted national initiatives to recruit and retain nurse providers, faculty, administrators, and researchers from diverse racial, cultural, and ethnic backgrounds.

I. Introduction

The growing consensus between consumers and the nursing community regarding health care reform provides a clear vision of how the nursing education system must now be re-directed—or re-formed—to serve the health needs of the people in the context of the twenty-first century. The changes in health care delivery that have occurred in the last decades, together with those now being proposed, magnify the challenges for a nursing education system undergoing its own changes.

The proposed reform of nursing education occurs as higher education itself faces significant challenges in regard to its relevance and accountability to the public it serves. The academic community, which was once the isolated domain of scholars, now includes practitioners, community and business leaders, and representatives of the foundation and public policy worlds as active partners in meeting its mission. As a result, the very nature of scholarship and the faculty role are being reconsidered.

Within this broader context, nursing education has initiated a series of its own fundamental reforms: re-formulating its mission, structure, and processes to include constituencies other than educators and disciplines other than nursing alone.

II. Nursing's Agenda for Health Care Reform

Nursing's Agenda for Health Care Reform—the nursing community's proactive position on how, where, and by whom health care should be delivered—ultimately depends for its success on a complementary stance in the educational sector. As a parallel to the fundamental changes in the proposed delivery system, long held beliefs about the mission, structure, and processes of nursing education are called into question by nursing's proposal for a consumer-driven, community-based system of primary care providers.

Nursing's Agenda calls for a new approach to delivery—taking health care to the consumer who will be an increasingly informed participant in decisions affecting his or her care. Health care services will be more usually delivered, for example, at work and school-based clinics. While hospitals and other institutions will still be significant components of the health care system, they will no longer be either the central focus or dominant influence. The consumer will now assume that position.

With the public's trust, nurses will also assume a new position within the proposed delivery system. Direct reimbursement for nursing services will position nurses, and make them even more directly accountable in the public eye. As nurses are encouraged to move into managed care arrangements, they will need different skills as administrators, managers, and coordinators of the care continuum in addition to the expertise necessary for providing primary care. Nursing's Agenda for Health Care Reform calls upon nurse providers to radically redefine their clinical practice, loyalties, political allies, and power nexus. No less is now expected of nursing education and nurse educators.

Clearly, the nature of the demand for nurses changes significantly from what has been the case until now. The proposed system is built upon the provider as a patient care manager—someone who combines the roles of patient advocate, knowledgeable advisor, triage officer, and access channel to the system; and someone who helps the patient and family choose wisely as they seek to assure their health and wellness.

III. NLN's Vision for Nursing Education Reform

Because the supply of nurses needed for the proposed delivery system differs from the current profile in both numbers and kind, nurse educators are faced with designing or modifying programs and curricula to assure that the nursing profession can deliver on the promises made within the reforms proposed. A community-based system calls on nurse educators to re-align their accountability away from institutions and agencies and toward populations. In so doing, the imperative of assuring that the graduates of their programs can deliver culturally competent care to the diverse populations who constitute those communities becomes more apparent;

as does the responsibility to recruit and retain individuals from diverse racial, cultural, and ethnic populations.

Therefore, as the alternative delivery system is in the process of being realized, the nursing education community is preparing to:

1. increase the numbers of advanced nurse practitioners in order to meet the need for primary care providers across the country;

2. reform all nursing education programs to assure that graduates are competent to function in a delivery system where:

   a. the individual and the family have primary responsibility for health care decisions;

   b. health and social issues are acknowledged as interactive and

   c. treatment effectiveness rather than the technologic imperative drives decisions.

3. re-define "nursing faculty" to include providers, re-socialize existing nursing faculty to the new roles appropriate for a community-based system, and re-form their knowledge base and repertoire of pedagogical skills.

IV. The Context for Reform

The Current Environment: In the educational sector the reforms needed in nursing education are as dramatic and as far-reaching as those proposed for the delivery system. Fortunately, the political climate for changes in nursing education is as favorable as the climate for change in the delivery sector because of recent trends in the higher education, health professions, and nursing education communities. Of the many significant departures from past educational practices, the following are among those with specific implications for how nursing education might be reformed in support of the Agenda.

1. *Higher Education.* First, the national movement toward greater public accountability for all educational programs has moved educators to be increasingly concerned with the outcomes of their programs and the expected or guaranteed competencies of their graduates. Second, the disturbing results of international comparisons among United States

graduates at both the secondary and post-secondary level have generated a national mood of reflection and introspection among educational policy makers. Third, there has been a broad-based national educational movement to reform curricula to those that are more socially relevant and particularly reflective of the diversity and plurality of local communities. Fourth, the increasingly high cost of a college education in both public and private institutions has led to the increased concerns for quality on the part of individual payers; and the public has begun to look with scrutiny on long-established practices such as the use of graduate students as faculty. Fifth, the economic exigencies of reduced resources challenge educational administrators. "Doing more with less" is the watchword as faculty develop new ways of teaching and advising. Many states have developed models of articulation between junior and senior colleges and some are paying greater attention to a "seamless" educational system that encompasses K through PhD. In other states all lower division courses are to be offered in community colleges.

2. *Education for Health Care Providers.*   Nursing education has engaged not only these issues of the broader educational community but those particular to the education of health care providers. First, technological advances that increase access to information call for a fundamental reorientation of the definitions and assumptions of both professionalism and education. The industrial model, which differentiated technical from professional work, is increasingly archaic and dysfunctional. In its place are models built around the individual as a knowledge worker within a system that places priority on primary health care. Differentiation among graduates solely on the basis of degrees is being replaced with differentiation on the basis of the competencies needed in various patient situations and expected from the graduates of particular programs.

Second, contemporary research in professional education points toward developing pattern recognition and innovative response to problems rather than to the mastery of any soon to be archaic content through a didactic pedagogy. The "art of thinking" is now considered an identical pattern, although in varying stages of development, whether the individual is a beginning or graduate student. Such research suggests a continuum rather than qualitative distinctions between the expected competencies of students and graduates of different programs.

Third, several recent commissions have identified an expanded range of competencies needed by tomorrow's health professionals. These competencies are increasingly not discipline specific, arguing more than ever before for a multidisciplinary approach, a broad and integrated knowledge base, and skills in collaboration, cooperation, and conflict resolution.

3. *Nursing Education.*   In addition, assumptions about nursing education have been similarly transformed by research and realities that question any arbitrary distinctions and outdated dichotomies between theory and practice. For example, recent research in the area of clinical decision making has led to a renewed recognition of the knowledge embedded in practice. Second, in contrast to the recent past, the profession now has a critical mass of clinicians with masters and post-masters education, prepared to serve as clinical faculty.

Furthermore, the era when the various pre-licensure nursing programs were distinct and self-contained entities has today been replaced by programmatic interaction and collaboration reinforced by state mandates for articulation agreements, a declining high school population, and the increasing numbers of second career students that characterize a national economy in transition. These new times lead to new ways of validating knowledge that are dependent neither on whether the courses are placed as an upper or lower division offering nor on their sequencing within a curriculum.

V. The Nursing Education Environment: Emerging Mission, Structure, and Processes

1. *The Emerging Mission.*   Increased public scrutiny matched with an intensified self-analysis has led nursing education to re-think its mission by re-thinking the traditional relationships among research, teaching, and community service. This triad has been at the heart of the university model first developed in eighteenth century Germany. What once served society well has become painfully out of touch with the complex issues of contemporary society. Research, teaching, and service rather than separate activities in the respective interest of the science, discipline, and professional community now need to assume new forms in the public interest and a more direct relationship to the community.

The mission of nursing education turns increasingly not only to the promotion of quality care by educating qualified practitioners but to the creation of linkages that will allow the educational projects of its faculty and students to actually provide services. Both research and learning can be expected to focus more on community health needs than has been the case.

2. *Emerging Community-Based Structures.*   While some of nursing education will continue to take place in academic settings, increasingly more will occur in the practice setting—but a practice setting within the community. Parallel to the increased emphasis on community-based delivery systems, nursing education programs will increasingly be structured so as to bring together the various constituencies concerned with the education of new nurses—the community, patients, current practitioners, students, business—in addition to the traditional faculty.

Educational experiences will be increasingly planned where people are—at home, in schools and work sites, in ambulatory settings, long-term care facilities, in shelters and community gathering places—as well as in hospitals. Given the growing difference from community to community throughout the country, nursing education programs may appear increasingly dissimilar reflecting the particular characteristics and specific needs of their locales.

Common to all programs, however, is the need to educate for the macro level of intervention rather than for micro individual situations, and for a greater authority, accountability, and responsibility and a lesser reliance on institutional authority and policies.

3. *Emerging Processes.*

a) *Curricular Reform.*   There is a generally acknowledged impetus to revise nursing curricula so that they are more accountable to the public. These calls for reforms include: a theoretical pluralism rather than any one "politically correct" approach; caring and humanitarianism as core values rather than the dominations of technology; and the centrality of the student-teacher relationship over esoteric scholarship.

Demographics argue for a major focus on care of the elderly and vulnerable populations as well as assurances that education provides a sensitivity and knowledge base that will inform care of diverse cultural and ethnic populations. Methods that increase students' sensitivity to all these populations must be sought, studied, and implemented.

Curricula at all levels will need to prepare graduates for management roles in all modalities of care wherein they will be able to work with assistive personnel, volunteers, and friends and families in new and complex ways. Graduates need to be prepared for managed care in the interest of clients, as contrasted with insurance companies or corporations, and be able to access and manage financial, technical, and human resources.

Calls for curricula innovations have also identified several areas for special attention such as:

1. Faculty-to-faculty and faculty-to-student relationships that are more egalitarian and characterized by cooperation and community building;

2. Special attention to the multicultural, multiracial and growing diversity of both individual and family lifestyles;

3. Incorporation of critique of the current health care system and an analysis of the present and future health needs of the population as the basis for transforming the health care system; and

4. Substantive contact with and participation by consumer populations, particularly those at health risk.

In addition, nursing education is working more closely than in recent history to match the needs of the emerging health care environment. Recent private studies, such as the Pew Commission, have identified trends within the larger environment that are of direct significance for education including:

1. Acute-care hospitals becoming a collection of intensive care units;

2. The increasing prevalence of self-care facilities and a move to greater consumer self-reliance;

3. An increasing public pressure for public disclosure, consumer information, and involvement;

4. A burgeoning home health industry;

5. The demographic shifts with accompanying expectations of elder care and chronic illness;

6. The adoption of clinical practice guidelines that create a more prescriptive practice while at the same time increase the opportunity for autonomous practice;

7. Limited financial, technical and human resources; and

8. Increased competition in the marketplace. While there is a tendency to approach curricular reform by focusing on which additional content and competencies ought to be included, this inevitably leads to missing the forest for the trees.

The most significant reform involves process—the changed relationship to information on the part of faculty, student, and health care consumer. Technology has democratized information and in the process shifted the points of access and control from the professional to the educated public. With this shift then, the focus of education turns from content to:

a. critical thinking,

b. skills in collaboration,

c. shared decision making,

d. social epidemiological viewpoint, and

e. analyses and interventions at the systems and aggregate levels.

b) *Faculty Reform.*   Critical to any discussion of educational reform is the recognition of the faculty as architects of curricula. Here, too, recent changes contribute to the receptive climate for educational reform especially as it relates to faculty scholarship. Nursing research has diversified considerably over the last two decades. With the exception of nurse anthropologists, nursing scholarship was once developed almost exclusively within the prevailing paradigm of the logical positivists. As it has matured, nursing scholarship has also broadened considerably. It now includes the work of qualitative methodologists, nurse philosophers and ethicists, historians, feminists, and most recently those working within Boyer's description of the "scholarship of application."

c) *The Scholarship of Application.*   There is a particular advantage for nursing faculty in Boyer's arguments for changing what is considered acceptable scholarship for appointment, promotion, and tenure within higher education. Of all the changes currently proposed, this has perhaps the greatest potential to reform higher education and advance Nursing's Agenda. Boyer argues for research studies more directly relevant to the broader social issues facing our society and our communities to replace the dominance of those studies of interest only to the particular discipline and its sub-specialists. He argues that for society's intellectual leadership to be more responsible and responsive it must address its attention to solving the concerns of daily living.

As a group, nursing faculty have demonstrated their abilities to be peer scholars within the academic community. Were they now to embrace the "scholarship of application" in addition to the more traditional definitions of scholarship, nursing faculty would be able to theoretically ground those projects within health care services provided as part of their teaching and their research. The cumulative effect will be a more inclusive view of what it means to be a scholar, and an intellectual pluralism that allows the faculty the orientation necessary for the curricula reform already discussed.

There is, however, one major exception to all this reform that must be addressed before any changes can be effected. Namely, that faculty teach what they know, and at this stage, the majority of faculty know the current health care system. Too few have been introduced, either by education, experience, or research to a consumer-driven, community-based primary health care system and even fewer are facile with their role as educators for such a system.

In addition, as lacking as these numbers seem to leave us, they under-report the need. We cannot assume that the community health we know and the community health nurses we have are what we need for the community health care that will emerge in the new system. Existing community and public health programs were developed for a different health care system than the one currently being proposed. The graduates of these programs, therefore, were prepared with the knowledge and skills needed for the soon to be reformed system. In the context of the significant delivery reforms being proposed, these educational programs themselves need to be rejuvenated, reformed, or relocated; and their graduates need additional post-graduate exposure.

Before curricular reform, then, comes faculty reform. As called for in the Secretary's Commission:

> We need nursing faculty who not only explore frontiers of new knowledge—but who also integrate ideas, connect thought to action, and inspire students . . .

Post-graduate programs are needed that will expand the expertise of current faculty and increase their facility in the following areas:

a) extra-institutional clinical sites,

b) population-based care,

c) cooperative relationships with consumers,

d) principles and practices of public health,

e) inner-disciplinary collaboration, and

f) new relationships to knowledge and technology.

Perhaps most importantly, faculty are urgently needed who are prepared to engage in research that will support and advance models that collapse the boundaries between education and practice, professional and patient, and those separating disciplines.

VI. Summary

Significant changes in nursing education are needed if the profession is to deliver on the promise embedded in Nursing's Agenda for Health Care Reform. In the past, nursing's focus on community-based care was philosophical for the many and actual only for the few who chose to specialize. Now, however, the Agenda for Health Care Reform is being advanced as nursing's alternative vision for health care delivery, and community-based care is increasingly the generalist's rather than the specialist's domain. Preparing all graduates of nursing education programs for community-based care, therefore, becomes the responsibility of all programs and all faculty. Perhaps in varying degrees, but a commonly shared responsibility, nonetheless.

REFERENCES

Boyer, E. L. Scholarship Reconsidered. Priorities of the Professorate. New Jersey, The Carnegie Foundation for the Advancement of Teaching, 1990.

National League for Nursing. (1991). *Nursing's Agenda for Health Care Reform*. New York: National League for Nursing Press.

"Innovative Curricula." Resolution Passed Unanimously by NLN Membership, 1989. Biennial Convention, Seattle, Washington.

Pew Health Professions Commission. Healthy America: Practitioners for 2005, An Agenda for Action for U.S. Health Professional Schools. Shugars, D. A., O'Neil, E. H., Bader, J. D. Durham: The Pew Health Professions Commission, October, 1991.

Other Books of Interest from NLN Press

Book Title	Pub. No.	Price	NLN Member Price
☐ Quality Imperatives in Long-Term Care: The Elusive Agenda *Edited by Ethel L. Mitty*	41-2440	25.95	22.95
☐ Mechanisms of Quality in Long-Term Care: Service and Clinical Outcomes	41-2382	10.50	10.50
☐ Indices of Quality in Long-Term Care: Research & Practice	20-2292	20.95	18.95
☐ Strategies for Long-Term Care	20-2231	16.50	16.50
☐ Review of Research in Nursing Education, Volume VI *By Lois Ryan Allen*	19-2544	27.95	24.95
☐ Living a Caring-Based Program *Edited by Anne Boykin*	14-2536	27.95	24.95
☐ Nursing as Caring: A Model for Transforming Practice *By Anne Boykin and Savina Schoenhofer*	15-2549	35.95	30.95
☐ Ways of Knowing and Caring for Older Adults *Edited by Mary M. Burke and Susan Sherman*	14-2541	29.95	26.95
☐ Gerontological Nursing: Issues and Opportunities for the 21st Century *Edited by Mary M. Burke and Susan Sherman*	14-2510	27.95	24.95